To Jill,
many Blessings
as you walk
through your cycles!
Ellen Kamhi
www.naturalnurse.com

CYCLES of LIFE

Also by Ellen Kamhi

The Natural Medicine Chest
coauthored with Eugene Zampieron, N.D.

Arthritis: The Alternative Medicine Definitive Guide
coauthored with Eugene Zamperion, N.D.

CYCLES of LIFE

Herbs and Energy Techniques For the Stages of a Woman's Life

Ellen Kamhi, Ph.D., R.N., H.N.C.
"The Natural Nurse"

M. Evans and Company, Inc.
New York

M. Evans and Company, Inc.
216 East 49th Street
New York, New York 10017

Library of Congress Cataloging-in-Publication Data

Kamhi, Ellen.
    Cycles of life : herbs and energy techniques for the stages of a woman's life / by Ellen Kamhi.
      p. cm.
    ISBN 0-87131-928-4
    1. Women—Health and hygiene. 2. Herbs—Therapeutic use. 3. Dietary supplements. I. Title.
    RA778 .K146 2001
    613'.04244—dc21   00-058703

Book design and typesetting by Rik Lain Schell

Printed in the United States of America

9 8 7 6 5 4 3 2 1

ATTENTION:

The information included in this book is for information purposes only. It is not intended to be used as a basis for self-treatment or as a substitute for professional medical care. The reader should consult a qualified health professional in regard to all symptoms, treatments, and dosage recommendations. Any reader taking prescription medication must be especially careful to seek professional medical attention before using any part of the remedies described in this book. The dosages discussed in this book are suggested dosages for adults, not children. The authors and publisher disclaim any responsibility for adverse effects related to the usage of any information presented in this book. Any application of the information contained in this book is at the reader's own discretion and risk.

I dedicate this book to the plants who have been my guides throughout the world, have sustained me, and have been my food and medicine. They continually bring beauty, comfort, excitement, contentment, and knowledge into my life.

Contents

Part III: Energy

List of Recipes

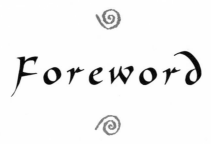

Foreword

As I finished reading the manuscript of this wonderful book, the third one of this prolific and wonderful healer, I felt a sense of motherly pride. For over ten years Ellen Kamhi has been and still is one of my most valuable associates. She is one of the most intellectually curious people I have ever met and has accumulated a vast array of medical knowledge which she simply and cleanly shares with her readers.

After attending Cornell and Rutgers Universities, Ellen spent several years living in a "palapa" (grass hut) in Mexico, apprenticing with an indigenous shaman. It was here that she discovered the efficacy of interacting with energy. She was able to experience first hand shamanic healers' astounding work, which often surpassed results that were obtained via the most advanced modern medicine. She continued her travels to Puerto Rico, Costa Rica, Jamaica, Spain, France, and Portugal, where she sought out and studied with natural healers trained in the lineage of their medicine people.

This book is full of very valuable and scientific information. I enjoyed it so much that when I reached the end I felt a longing for more. In *Cycles of Life* Ellen Kamhi displays vast knowledge about herbal and "energetic" medicine. Her approach gives a new perspective on combining Western medical scientific research with the millennia of human experience. As she herself states, her quest for understanding of the medicinal properties of herbs began a long time ago—when she was only twelve years old. This journey has continued all of her life, with no end in sight. Ellen has had a most fascinating life. She has learned from the wisdom of native medicine; wisdom that goes back to the beginning of civilization.

Undoubtedly you will have the privilege of taking advantage of her personal journey and years of exposure to scientific integrative medicine. She wonderfully explains the female physiology while giving the reader prescriptions for natural remedies to correct both small and large imbalances. The first part of the book is, in fact, a very valuable cavalcade through the female cycle of life and how to manage its various steps—including herbs, visualization, music, and various natural modes of healing. Dr. Kamhi's experience as a midwife and an herbalist shines through as she gives superb advice on what to do during pregnancy, birth, and lactation. Her expertise extends through to the latter part of a woman's cycle, namely the transition from the fertility stage to the "wise woman" stage.

The second part of the book affords us with a more detailed explanation of natural remedies and strategies of healing. Applied herbal medicine is the largest human clinical study ever. Cave men and women used their instincts, just as animals do, and tried countless natural products to heal themselves. The results were passed on from one generation to the next, with further refinements. Until the advent of pharmaceutical medicine, herbs and other natural interventions were the true healers. Fortunately, we have entered a new era of rediscovery of the collective wisdom of our ancestors, and are making good use of it.

Ellen Kamhi has had the good fortune of experiencing this wisdom first hand. Here she brings together the plethora of research and scientific background available in today's herbal pharmacopeia.

The part of this book I personally found to be of greatest interest was about biological rhythms. Ellen Kamhi has the ability to interface with the world's most brilliant people in the field of energy medicine. You will—as I have—benefit enormously from being able to tap into this network. Her information on biological rhythms is revolutionary yet easy to read. It includes information on the effect of "geophysical" factors on our physiology and suggests that we can harness these geophysical forces to use them to our advantage whenever possible. Dr. Kamhi empowers the reader with the tools for self-choice and self-determination.

I am sure you will find *Cycles of Life: Herbs and Energy Techniques for the Stages of a Woman's Life* as fascinating, useful, and full of valuable and practical information as I have.

Serafina Corsello, M.D.

Acknowledgments

This book was truly a labor of love. I thank G-d every day for my ongoing journey in the field of natural medicine. It has brought the light of true healing to myself, family, friends, associates, and patients throughout the decades. Blessings always to my parents, Sondra and Julius Kamhi, and to my children, Titus and Ali, and Brenda. To my business partner and cofounder of Natural Alternatives—Health Education and Multi-Media Services, Eugene Zampieron, N.D., for his major contributions, both written and photographic, towards this book; I give my eternal thanks and blessings to our association. I would like to send a special thanks to the illustrators Ann Rothan, Renee Joseph, Ehren Joseph, and MATT, and the photographers Eugene Zampieron, Tom Hammang, Norm Suhu, Walt Carr, and Mark Raskin. To Michael Berman, my life partner, who literally sat next to me during the research and typing of this entire manuscript; I send my love. To you, the reader, blessings on your path to herbal and energetic knowledge; may the truth and wisdom of nature abound!

Introduction

I am woman . . . blatantly and repeatedly confronted with my changes; hormonal harmonics stirring moon time visions, ovulatory oracles, pre-menstrual crazies, orgasmic knowings, birth ecstasies, breast feeding bliss, menopausal moods. . . .
—Susan Weed, *Healing Wise*

Women in every corner of the globe use herbs as they progress through the cycles of life. They rely on plants to nourish; to heal; to protect; to lift spirits; to give solace, strength, joy, and hope; and to provide every conceivable system of support to both the selves and the cells of women everywhere. Energy healing—the interlacing of the human psyche, nature, and the subtle eminence that permeates all matter—has been used to balance and support the healing realm since the dawn of history.

Herbal medicine is as old as humanity itself! Ancient people used many techniques to determine which plants were safe and helpful for various conditions. Trial and error played a major role. Since many plants are poisonous, some early herbalists got sick or even died during initial trials of plant medicines. A safer method was found when our ancestors noticed that animals used "instinctual dousing." Many creatures consume certain plants only when they have a specific health condition—you can observe this behavior in cats and dogs. They eat grass when they have an upset stomach; this will often cause them to vomit, relieving the condition. Folkloric healers to this day rely on dousing techniques.

Indiginous healers—referred to as shamans—claim to obtain information about plant medicine through communication with the divine in a dream state or during communion with the spirit world. They also find clues left by the Creator—"holy signatures"—on the plants, which provide hints on how the plant might best be used as medicine. The Doctrine of Signatures is a similar modern teaching that claims plants often contain clues, which may be part of their appearance, growing habits, or other attributes, that reflect a medicinal use for that plant. A good example is Ginkgo biloba: its leaves and fruit resemble the human brain. Scientific research has shown that Ginkgo can improve brain function.

As knowledge of plant medicine grew, it was passed down from generation to generation, archived in oral or written form depending on the culture. Throughout the world, women were guardians of herbal knowledge. This role was sometimes revered, but often led to persecution. During the European Middle Ages, wise weed women and midwives kept herbal traditions intact. In fact, one of the most famous of the women healers of this era is revered by the Roman Catholic Church: St. Hildegard of Bingen (1098–1179) was a gifted herbalist who authored *Liber Simplicis Medicine*, in which she discussed hundreds of herbal medicines. Wise women like Hildegard were often the only health care resource available for poor people.

Unfortunately, however, not all healers were granted such respect. The male-dominated medical aristocracy brought a claim to the medieval church that women who healed with herbs and energy techniques were using a form of satanic power. The church supported the medical profession, in effect outlawing herbal and energy medicine as practiced by women. The sanction for practicing thousands of years of human tradition was death, often by being burned alive at the stake. This policy was followed for over two hundred years—many thousands of women were killed, and millions more were deprived of health care. Yet in spite of all this persecution, the wise women traditions continue today.

My own journey into natural healing began when I was twelve

years old. I had a severe injury after falling off a horse, and the doctors felt that surgery would be needed. I decided to go to the local library and research to see if there were any alternative suggestions. I was truly amazed by what was available! After scratching just a little bit below the surface I was able to uncover all kinds of information about using natural therapies to heal an injured lower back. These included foods; energy techniques such as meditation, hands-on healing, and magnets; lifestyle changes; nutritional supplements; and plant medicines. I had to order many things through the mail, since there weren't any health food stores where I was living at the time. Although I was truly impressed by how well I was able to heal by following the natural suggestions I had discovered, I was also dismayed at the lack of interest displayed by the medical authorities. They dismissed my recovery without surgery as merely a "coincidence." They claimed that I had experienced a "spontaneous remission" totally unrelated to my dabbling in "that old folklore stuff." My own understanding of the term *coincidence* is a little different. It means two or more simultaneous events occurring together and intersecting in a deeply meaningful way. I *knew* the natural therapies had indeed cured my problem, and this event started me on a lifelong quest that continues to this day. I am forever grateful for this knowledge, which has helped me, my family, and thousands of patients throughout the years deal with health imbalances.

As spiral cycles continue, like nautilus shells, in ever intertwining paths throughout time and space, so we are witness to the modern-day return of the medicinal use of herbs as a recognized healing art, and energy healing as the medicine of the future. Science is substantiating what tribal healers have known for centuries; that plants and energy healing make good medicine.

how to Use
This Book

As we explore the use of herbs and energy techniques in healing, remember the cycles we are all a part of: our own internal monthly cycle, our seasons, our community, our planet. *Cycles, cycles,* women's lives run on cycles—moon cycles, monthly cycles, hormone cycles, love cycles . . . infant, toddler, child, pre-teen, adolescent, young woman, lover, mate, mother, friend, grandmother, crone . . . Plant medicines have the uncanny ability to bring balance to a sometimes out-of-balance life. This capacity is referred to as *adaptogenic.* Red raspberry leaf is a women-friendly herb that has this ability. It can act to either relax or tone the uterus. Although science can prove that specific active constituents found in red raspberry leaves can be documented to have this dual effect, all of science cannot yet explain *how* the chemicals "know" which opposing effect an individual women needs. Although science teaches us that all things can be explained, more ancient, time-tested belief systems repeatedly remind us that there are still many mysteries.

Plant medicine and energy healing fit into these mystery traditions. In this book we will take a journey through the cycles of Llife—the labyrinth that all women walk through: *Menarche,* as a young woman reaches her first menstruation; *The Menstrual Years,* with issues such as PMS, cysts, and fibroids; *Fertility,* both desired and not; and *Menopause,* a door to "the golden years."

First, in Part I, we'll discuss our forever "raging" hormones, how they work, and what problems may occur if they are out of balance. As we go through each cycle we'll discuss some of the important issues women face, along with how to best balance focused areas of health and wellness using therapies like foods, mental and physical exercises, and energy techniques. My recommendations for herbal therapies that I have suggested to my patients for over thirty years are included for each condition. In-depth information about herbs in **boldface** type can be found in Part II, which is a basic *materia medica*. This list of thirty-four herbs commonly used for women's wellness includes background information and specific instructions on how to use them, including dosage. Part III covers several energy healing techniques, including circadian rhythms, the effect of music on hormones, and essence remedies. Finally, we'll conclude with a symptom cross-reference section, which you can use to quickly access information on the best herbs to use for different health imbalances.

Now join me on a journey through *The Cycles of Life!*

Part I

The Life Cycles

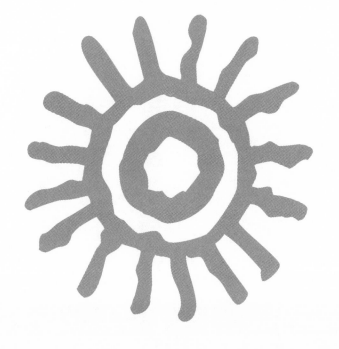

hormones

Hormonal Harmonics

There is an intricate interplay and balance between many hormones, each having its own cycle within a woman's body. Listed below you will find the major ones that are involved in the female reproductive cycle.

THE MAJOR HORMONES

Estrogen is known as the "female hormone" because it is responsible for the development of female secondary sex characteristics such as breast development. Estrogen is not just one hormone, but a group of hormones. The three main varieties of estrogen are estrone (E-1), estradiol (E-2), and estriol (E-3). Some types of estrogen are more aggressive than others and are linked to many health problems, including mild annoyances such as occasional breast tenderness to serious illnesses such as cancer. Aggressive estrogens can be tempered or "opposed" by milder estrogens,

1

which fit into the same *estrogen receptor sites* and thereby oppose the action of the aggressive estrogens. This is how *phytoestogens* from plants work. Many health problems linked to the hormonal harmonics that are orchestrated in a woman's body can be linked to "unopposed estrogen," which in turn can be caused by an over-burdened liver; low progesterone levels; heightened aggressive estrogen levels due to a diet high in pesticides, herbicides, and toxic chemicals; or toxic emotional states. These problems include premenstrual syndrome (PMS), polycystic ovaries and breasts, endometriosis, irregular menstruation, infertility, menopausal complaints, and most other conditions that are related to hormone levels.

Testosterone is thought of as the "male hormone" because it acts to develop male traits, such as a deep voice and beard. The truth is, both men and women have estrogen and testosterone, with the proportion of each differing depending on the person's sex. In women, testosterone is produced in the ovaries, adrenal glands, and liver. It is interesting to note that the area of the brain that contains testosterone receptors is involved with love and lust. Testosterone in low amounts is important in women to maintain a heightened libido, and insure muscle mass. If levels of testosterone are too high, it can cause conditions such as excess facial hair growth, acne, and polycystic ovaries.

Progesterone is another hormone that is intricately connected to the female cycle (although men also have some progesterone). The word progesterone is from the latin *progestin* which means "before pregnancy." It is the hormone that maintains pregnancy, and is naturally found in high levels during that time as well as during the second half of the menstrual cycle, between ovulation and menstruation. Dr. Serafina Corsello explains in detail in *The Ageless Woman* the beneficial effects of progesterone that tend to go unrecognized by mainstream medicine. "Progesterone is involved in a wide range of important physiologic activities. It is necessary for the proper binding of thyroid hormone to the tissues, and it modulates glucose metabolism. It reduces blood clotting and water retention, promotes cell division, and stabilizes our moods." Progesterone offsets unopposed estrogen. It is the ratio between progesterone and estrogen that is the most important factor in decreasing the many physiological problems associated with unopposed estrogen.

FSH (Follicle Stimulating Hormone) and LH (Luteinizing Hormone) are messenger hormones released by the pituitary gland. Early in the menstrual cycle, estrogen levels are very low stimulating the hypothalamus (a part of the brain) to release a messenger called GnRH. GnRH (Hypothalamic Gonadotrophin Releasing Hormone) in turn stimulates the pituitary to release FSH. FSH is responsible for the development of the follicles, which are sacs that contain the egg. The average woman is born with two million eggs. Starting with menarche, one (or occasionally more) eggs are released each month. The follicle secretes estrogen as it develops and blood levels of estrogen begin to peak. In response to the increasing amounts of estrogen, FSH levels drop. The estrogen levels continue to rise in this follicular phase, stimulating the uterine lining to thicken.

At midcycle, there is a LH surge. The surge of LH completes the maturation of the dominant follicle. In a short time, the egg will be ready to be released from the follicle (ovulation). Once ovulation occurs, the empty follicle is termed *corpus luteum*, a yellow fatty area that is formed from the sac that previously housed the egg. The secretion of estrogen continues, and now progesterone is secreted from the corpus luteum, beginning the *luteal phase*. It is at this juncture that fertilization of the egg is possible. If fertilization occurs, along with implantation of the fertilized egg in the lining of the uterus, the levels of these hormones accelerate. If pregnancy is not achieved, the levels fall and a new cycle begins, starting with the sloughing off of the no longer needed enhanced uterine lining. This is the menstrual flow. The level of each hormone sends a signal between the brain and ovary with great intricacy. It is an awesome system (see the chart on the following page), but if any of the hormones are out of sync for any reason, problems can ensue.

The Female Cycle [1]

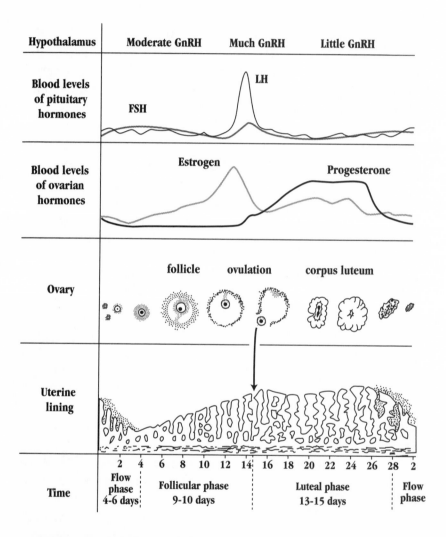

Reprinted with permission from *The Ageless Woman* by Serafina Corsello, M.D.

Prolactin is another hormone that is important to a woman's body. The normal function of prolactin is to regulate milk flow in a nursing mother. During this time, prolactin inhibits the secretion of LH, FSH, and progesterone. In non-nursing women, both low progesterone levels and high prolactin levels are found in women who have delayed or inhibited ovulation, infertility, endometriosis, PMS, cystic ovaries, fibrocystic breasts, fibroid, tumors and endometriosis. Prolactin is produced by the pituitary gland, but when a woman's body is under stress—whether it be chemical, physical, psychological or emotional—lymphocytes (white blood cells) will also produce prolactin. Prolactin levels can be further elevated due to low levels of magnesium, vitamin B-6, and disturbed digestion.

Phytosterols—Plant Hormones

The term *phytosterol* refers to chemical compounds found in plants that are often, but not always, very similar to steroidal hormones found in humans. Herbs and plant foods high in phytosterols have been used by humans for millennia as medicines for hormone-related health issues such as menstruation, fertility, and childbirth—long before chemical analysis existed! Research has shown that phytosterols seem to have a protective effect on human tissue, such as soybean's ability to decrease the incidence of breast cancer.[2] The phytosterols fit into estrogen binding sites, thereby inhibiting more aggressive estrogens from binding there; agressive estrogens that could initiate a toxic cascade leading to cancer or other diseases. There are also many plants that are claimed to have estrogenic or hormonal effects, but chemical analysis indicates that no phytosterols are present. Further investigations have revealed that these plants contain other chemicals that can fit into estrogen receptor sites, and have an estrogenic effect on organs or body systems. The chemicals in these plants may have other effects such as increased circulation or muscle relaxation.

Listed below are some of the well-known phytosterols along with plants that contain them. A few plants actually contain compounds that are almost identical to estrogen found in humans, including *estriol, estradiol,* and *estrone.* These plants, when used as food and medicine, can profoundly influence the hormone levels in the human system.

B-sitosterol—red clover, saw palmetto
Diosgenen—wild yam
Estriol—licorice, green bean
Estradiol—hops, green beans
Estrone—green beans, dates, pomegranates

CHAPTER TWO

Menarche
Ovulatory Oracles

RITUALS

As a young woman reaches the age of her first menstruation or menarche, there are changes that occur in her body and mind that can be quite overwhelming. There are many changes that herald this entry into a change of life. Physical changes are obvious, such as growth of pubic hair and breast development, but equally important are the emotional and psychological changes that accompany this important phase of growth and development. Ancient societies have always used herbs and ceremony to aid in this time of transition.

In indigenous societies, the beginning of the menses is marked by recognition and fanfare. An example of this is the Sun Ceremony celebrated by the Apache Nations People. This ritual occurs during the summer season following a young girl's first period. A time of withdrawal from the group is accompanied by special foods, chants, prayers, and making of ceremonial garments. On the day of the cer-

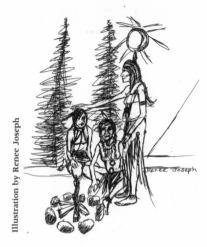

Illustration by Renee Joseph

emony an older woman (usually not the girl's mother) acts as a liaison between the young initiate and Changing Woman—the entity who brings the girl into her newfound womanhood, makes her spiritually strong, and prepares her for a long life. The entire group celebrates this important transition and recognizes the change that has occurred. The new life now carries increased power, along with increased responsibilities.[3]

A more recent ritual is the Jewish tradition of the Bat Mitzvah, previously celebrated only for young men as the Bar Mitzvah. During the ceremony the thirteen-year-old officially takes on the responsibilities of adulthood. The parent is symbolically released from the "karma" of the actions of the child, so to speak. Any consequences, either positive or negative, caused by the child's actions are no longer the parents' spiritual responsibility.

However, in modern America there seems to be a lack of support to young women going through this important transition. In particular, there is no universal rite of passage from childhood to womanhood sanctioned by American culture. A vast majority of modern girls are thrust into the experience of donning a new body, as well as a new psyche, without the benefit of any kind of transitional recognition. About the most they say is "I got my period," and somehow they are expected to act more grown up. For one thing, they probably already know about such things as sanitary napkins, tampons, and even over-the-counter birth control and pregnancy tests. These are now common knowledge for everyone (even younger brothers) due to the public proliferation of this kind of information through the onslaught of mass media. Even though these messages are so prolific, there is no spiritual or emotional recognition of this special cycle in a young woman's life.

USING HERBS FOR MODERN RITUAL

Wildcrafting—actually going out into the field to pick your own herbs—can be an initiation ritual for adolescents. It is a grounding and restorative adventure, and can offset the overstimulation of artificial wavelengths of light, food, and energy that we are all bombarded with in the twenty-first century. I regularly lead weed walks to identify wild edible and medicinal plants, through my organization, Natural Alternatives, and in association with the Cornell Cooperative Extension and the Nature Conservancy. Join me or find an herbalist or naturalist in your own locality to lead the way! If you prefer a milder adventure, stalk the aisles of your local health food store, or visit an e-commerce online store to locate these herbs in already prepared tinctures, extracts, or capsules.

CAUSES OF IMBALANCE DURING MENARCHE

Early Onset of menstruation can have negative effects. Although textbooks still list the average age as thirteen to sixteen years old, most girls in the United States start their period much younger, as early as nine or ten. It is well documented that early onset is linked to an increased risk of breast and uterine cancer.[4] Another problem with early onset is the emotional and psychological pressures that come along with sexual maturation starting too soon. Peer pressure, combined with biological urges, can open the door to promiscuity at an early age, before the young girl has enough life experience to understand the ramifications and risks associated with the "joy of sex."

Xenoestrogens are estrogen-like compounds that are highly toxic. Xenoestrogens are one of the major causes of irregularities in the smooth initiation of menarche. They are found throughout the environment as by-products of pesticides, herbicides, and synthetic hormones routinely fed to animals, which are stored in the animals' fat and transferred to people who eat them. Xenoestrogens also come from petrochemicals and plastics, the coating inside canned foods, and even baby bottles! Once inside the body xeno-estrogens can be strong carcinogens. They compete with more mild forms of estrogen for specific receptor cites, and play havoc with the normal mechanisms of the reproductive cycle.

Visual Sexual Stimulation is overabundant in modern America. There is virtually no way for a young girl, or anyone else for that matter, to avoid viewing sexually suggestive material that abounds on TV, movies, the Internet, and even on roadside bill-boards! Viewing these images actually stimulates the release of sex hormones, which may speed up sexual maturation.

HEALTH ISSUES DURING MENARCHE

There are many health issues that are common to young women as they go through the life cycle of menarche. Whether menarche is "premature," or occurs at the "normal" age, herbs can be a wonderful support for the tumultuous changes that occur.

Nutrition

The need for good nutrition is of utmost importance at the time of menarche due to a young woman's rapid growth and develop-ment. Unfortunately, the tendency to eat out with friends also increases, and the trend is to frequent fast-food places. Even if a young woman cannot be wholly convinced to eat healthy, herbs can be used to augment nutritional requirements.

> HERBS FOR NUTRITIONAL SUPPORT: **Sea vegetables, nettle, green foods**

Menarche

Emotions

Emotional stability is often challenged during menarche. Adolescence is a time of emotional turmoil. Crying bouts are common as feelings of doubt about self-worth become paramount. Peer approval is increasingly important and young women are extremely sensitive about being accepted by "the crowd." Friendship with boys loses some of its innocence as puppy love and crushes become part of the social scene. Defining a new adult personality can be a shaky experience, similar to taking the first steps as a toddler. It's not uncommon for the teenage girl to regress to some preadolescent behaviors, such as thumbsucking.

> HERBS FOR EMOTIONAL STABILITY: There are several herbs that can help to smooth this transition as the blossoming woman emerges from the little girl. **Chamomile** and **rose buds** used as teas, extracts, or capsules can gently calm the mood. **Bach flower remedies** are extremely helpful, too.

Acne

Acne is not limited to menarche, but is most prevalent during this time. The skin eruptions associated with acne closely mirror the tumultuous emotional and hormonal changes that accompany this transitional cycle. Natural protocols for acne must recognize the interplay between spiritual, physical, and emotional factors that all play a part in the cause and treatment of this condition. Although much of conventional medicine does not recognize the role that diet and food allergies have in skin conditions, most natural healers believe there is a direct correlation.

NUTRITION FOR ACNE: It is wise to focus on a diet low in milk products, processed wheat, and animal fat; and high in organic leafy green vegetables, whole grains, and omega-3 oils such as flaxseed and hemp oils.

HERBS FOR ACNE: Herbal remedies for acne fall under the category of herbs known as alteratives. Doctors of the Eclectic school around 1900 referred to alteratives as "blood and lymphatic cleansers." Alteratives are non-toxic herbs that assist the organs of detoxification and elimination (liver, bowels, kidneys, skin, lungs, and connective tissue) by removing deleterious substances such as environmental toxins as well as those generated internally by the body. Alterative herbs useful for acne are **dandelion**, **burdock** and **red clover**. A commercially available alterative is *Alteratonic*. (See www.naturesanswer.com.)

ACNE SKIN SALVE

Squeeze about 2 inches of **aloe vera** gel (available in health food stores) into your palm. Add two or three drops of **tea tree oil** and mix into the gel. Use this directly on skin for soothing and clearing acne. Washing the skin twice a day with *Grandpa's Pine Tar Soap* is also helpful for acne and many other skin conditions.

For the recipe for ***ACNE BURDOCK COMPRESS,*** see page 96.

Digestive Problems

Constipation, indigestion, and flatulence are common during menarche. Acne is often accompanied by imbalanced bowel function. The hormones that govern the release of digestive enzymes are part of the changing cycle young women experience.

NUTRITION FOR DIGESTIVE PROBLEMS: Digestion can be aided greatly by decreasing the consumption of fried foods, processed foods, and dairy products; and increasing fresh fruits, vegetables, and whole grains. Probiotics (beneficial bacteria), such as acidophilus and bifidus preparations (available in any health food store) are of great value for reestablishing a healthy digestive system.

HERBS FOR DIGESTION: **Chamomile, ginger, licorice,** and peppermint are herbs that can aid digestion. **Cascara sagrada** is a useful herbal laxative.

Menstruation

Period irregularities are common during menarche. However, if nutrition and emotions are attended to, many problems will rectify themselves. Herbs can help with a rough beginning of the menstrual cycle.

HERBS TO BALANCE PERIOD IRREGULARITIES: **Chaste tree berry, black cohosh, Dong quai,** and **red raspberry leaf**.

Menarche is a cycle experienced by the young. Usually, if given the right nutrients, the body will overcome imbalances and move smoothly into the next cycle—*The Menstruating Years.*

CHAPTER THREE

the
Menstruating Years

Moontime Mysteries

I had some difficulty naming this chapter. First I thought of "Womanhood," but all phases of life can be so titled. Womanhood is certainly not over when we enter menopause. Then I thought of "the Childbearing Years," but many woman have a totally full life without going through childbearing and raising families. So here we have "the Menstruating Years," which accurately describes the cycle of life we will discuss in this section. This time of life is a very busy one for most women. For perhaps the first time in history, the boundaries between the sexes in terms of role model expectations have been shattered. Women are no longer relegated to a life of "domestic bliss," pregnancy, child care, and homemaking. Many women opt to include all these things, however, along with a professional life. The fact remains that women who work still carry the bulk of responsibility for childcare, cooking, and cleaning, even if they work the same number of hours as their spouses do.[5] This condition is often referred to as "Super Woman," and stands as the perceived ideal for today's modern woman. The fact that women bleed monthly is considered unimportant in modern society. However, this was not always the case.

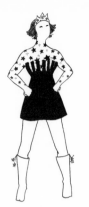

Illustration by Ann Rothan

RITUALS FOR THE MENSTRUATING YEARS

Menstrual Mysteries—Moon Time Visions

In civilizations around the world and throughout history the monthly bleeding time was widely recognized as a special time. Menstruating women were separated from society through various methods. In the Eastern practice of yoga it is suggested that women refrain from inverted yoga postures, such as the shoulder stand, during menstruation. According to the Jewish faith, women do not sleep in the same bed as their husbands during this time of the month. When the menstrual flow ends they enter a special sanctified ritual bath before rejoining the nuptial bed. Other societies actually provide special huts or sleeping quarters for women during their moontime. The moon is used as a symbol for women and their monthly cycles because the moon's cycle of twenty-eight days closely matches the menstrual cycle. In some cultures women were believed to possess special powers during that time of the month, and were often excluded from routine events. There were special herbs, baths, prayers, and rituals that women indulged in during "those days."

All this special recognition and separation may seem archaic in today's modern world, where we pop a Motrin, shove in a tampon, and fulfill the pretense that "these days" are like any other. Advertisements from Madison Avenue focus on how we can cover up the odor, use a thin, non-showing pad, and, in general, breeze through with as little discomfort as possible. However, how much is actually lost by this modern attitude? Although it may make us more able to fully function in a man's world, what of the loss of mystical power, special privilege, and, yes, perhaps a few days to rest, relax, reflect, regroup, and recuperate from the stresses of everyday life?

A woman's moontime is still steeped in mystery. Psychic powers and the ability to see between the veils are potentiated. Seeing between the veils is understood by various mystery school teachings as the ability to see through the layers of illusion that are presented to us as "reality." These teachings seek an understanding of the true meaning of existence. Here is a ritual you can use to honor the sacredness of "those days."

Earth-Bonding to Open the Dream Time Doors

Arrange to spend time alone during your period. Get a baby-sitter, take some sick days, visit a friend (especially one who lives out in the country), whatever it takes. This ritual is especially helpful if you are involved in a confusing life transition. Spend the first day alone just resting. Avoid television, radio, or Internet. Sleep or nap all you want. Do some gentle breathing and stretching. Take time to write both your long-term and immediate life goals in a journal. Investigate your inner self through the use of Essence Remedies (see page 172).

On the second day prepare for an earth-bonding ritual. Find a secluded spot in the woods. (If this is not possible, fill a shallow container with earth.) Gather together some of the following herbs: sage, red beet root, angelica, dandelion, scented geranium, lavender, or any other herbs that you feel attracted to. Bring a red and white candle—red to reflect the power of your blood, white to honor your spiritual intention. Mix all herbs together in a bowl. Add a few drops of lavender oil. Light the herb oil mixture. Light the candles. Rub angelica oil (dong quai oil) on your lower abdomen over the area of your uterus. Write a prayer or intention clearly on white unlined paper. As you focus on your intention, burn the paper in the bowl of herbs while you allow your menstrual flow to go onto the earth, either the forest floor or the earth

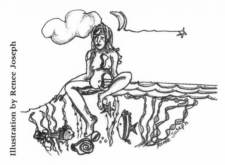

Illustration by Renee Joseph

in your container. Imagine the true grounding that is taking place between you and Mother Earth. Feel her strength enter you. No man can have this experience. It is the mystery of woman, who bleeds without dying. Allow yourself to integrate whatever emotions this ritual initiates, be it calmness, pain, joy, or sorrow. Some women prefer to do this ritual near a natural body of water, entering the water world to perform the bonding. This experience is enriching in the development of true female energy. Feel the special separation that allows women to open the dream time doors during the menstrual flow.

After your earth-bonding take some time to reintegrate back into normal life. Rub your skin with sea salt and then shower. Put on different clothes. Carry your renewed power back with you into daily life.

DETOXIFICATION

Before we discuss specific health issues that concern women during the menstruating years, we need to introduce one of the first steps that we often recommend to women of all ages who are having health problems, including those linked to hormones—detoxification, or detox. Detoxification is a process widely recognized throughout history as a method to rest and heal the body. There are many methods of detoxification. Most employ some degree of fasting to allow the digestive system to eliminate toxins that have accumulated over time. This type of fasting does not involve starvation. Hormones cycle monthly in the female body. The detoxification systems need to be functioning optimally in order to break down these hormones. An overabundance of certain forms of estrogen and other hormones, including prolactin, lead to a variety of female health issues including PMS, infertility, and cystic and fibroid conditions. Here we will outline a detoxification program that will help to clear the liver, kidneys, skin, and bowels—the main organs of detoxification. Many women find that following this program for a week, two to three times per year, keeps them free from all symptoms. An added bonus to detoxification is natural weight control along with increased energy, an elevated mental/emotional state, and a renewed sense of self-awareness and self-control.

Preparing for Detoxification

Prepare for detoxification by gathering all the herbs and foods that you will need beforehand, so you can relax and enjoy the process. Cook a full pot of Detoxifying Vegetable Soup (see recipe below) . Be sure all cooking utensils are *not* aluminum. Stainless steel or glass cookware is a good choice.

Try a mini-fast along with herbs to cleanse the bowels, reduce constipation, support the liver, and increase flow of lymph fluid.

DETOXIFYING VEGETABLE SOUP

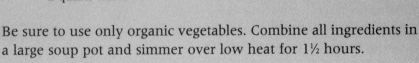

1 onion, peeled and chopped
1 head cabbage, chopped
2 cloves garlic, peeled and chopped
2 carrots, chopped
2 celery stalks, trimmed and chopped
1 bunch parsley, chopped
5 kale leaves, chopped
2 sheets nori sea vegetable
4 pieces okra, trimmed and chopped
1 cup uncooked brown rice
pinch Bragg's Amino Acids
2 quarts water

Illustration by Ann Rothan

Be sure to use only organic vegetables. Combine all ingredients in a large soup pot and simmer over low heat for 1½ hours.

Mini-Fasting

For three days eat as much of the Detoxifying Vegetable Soup as you like. Drink as much water and herb tea as you want. Any two fruits can be included as snacks, but are optional. You can continue past the three days for up to seven days if you prefer. Also use

green foods mixed in water, and any green vegetable juice, up to four glasses a day.

When you end your mini-fast do not eat any fried, processed, or sugar laden foods for at least another two days. Avoiding these foods *altogether* is the best choice. This will give your bowels and liver a rest. They will then be better prepared to break down excess estrogen by your next period.

Colon Detox

If you experience constipation during detoxification try **cascara sagrada** along with ¼ teaspoon psyllium seeds in 8 ounces of water twice per day. You may find it helpful to do an enema on any day that you fail to have a bowel movement during detoxification.

Liver Detox

The liver is an important organ of detoxification. Its job is to filter out impurities from the blood. When it becomes overburdened through the accumulation of toxins, it can no longer break down excess hormones efficiently. That is why it is important to support and cleanse the liver. Herbs can aid the liver in this process.

> HERBS FOR THE LIVER: **Dandelion, burdock, Ho Shu Wu, licorice root, milk thistle.**

Lymph System Detox

The lymph fluid flows through the entire body and bathes all internal tissues in nutrient rich fluids. It also picks up waste products to flush them out of the body. Lymph nodes are located in various areas of the body, such as the armpits, groin, and throat, to help filter these impurities out of the lymph fluid. Swollen glands felt under the neck or tender breasts before the period are examples of lymph nodes that are overburdened with fluid and waste products. An extreme condition can lead to breast cancer with lymph node involvement. Detoxification makes the lymph fluid less viscous (thick), and allows it to flow more easily throughout all body tissues, placing less pressure on the lymph nodes. Please note, however, that during the detoxification process, the lymph nodes may temporarily become tender because the body is dumping out a lot of waste. The suggestions which follow help to support the lymph system.

HERBS FOR THE LYMPH SYSTEM: Cleavers, **red clover, nettle**, pokeroot. (Although pokeroot is the ultimate lymphatic cleanser, it can be toxic and should be used under the guidance of a health care professional. However, you can use it safely as a homeopathic remedy called *Phytolacca*.)

OTHER USEFUL LYMPHATIC CLEANSERS:
Massage
Jumping on a mini-trampoline
Dry skin brushing
Castor oil pack

DRY SKIN BRUSHING

Purchase a dry skin brush made of natural bristles or a loofah sponge. *Before* getting into the shower or bath, brush the skin with long strokes, using enough pressure to feel some light friction. Brush towards the heart. This stimulates the lymphatic system and also brushes off dead skin cells.

For the recipe for **CASTOR OIL PACK,** see page 100.

The castor oil pack applied externally to breasts, uterus, or any other area where you experience cysts, discomfort, hard tissues, spasms, or pain can be one of the most helpful therapies available. It increases circulation to the area, softens tissues, and can actually pull toxins out through the skin. Adding thuja oil (red cedar) and phytolacca oil (pokeroot) increases the effectiveness of the castor oil pack.

CYCLES OF LIFE

HEALTH ISSUES DURING
THE MENSTRUATING YEARS

There are many health issues that are linked to the menstrual cycle. These include yeast infections, PMS, and cystic and fibroid conditions like fibrocystic breasts, ovarian cysts, and endometriosis. Fertility issues such as contraception, infertility, pregnancy, and nursing will be discussed in the next chapter.

Yeast Infections

Yeast infections are most commonly caused by an overgrowth of the yeast organism *Candida albicans.* Yeast infections can be experienced as a local infection in the vagina, or can become systemic, where the growth of yeast occurs in other organs throughout the body, as well as in the bloodstream. Candida is actually a normal part of the flora found in the intestines and vagina. It becomes a troublesome vaginal infection when it begins to grow profusely, causing a white, cottage cheese–like discharge along with uncomfortable itching. Yeast infections are two and a half times more prevalent than twenty years ago. Systemic yeast infections can be detected by an anti-candida antibody blood titer test ordered by a physician. A darkfield blood analysis, where a drop of blood is viewed under a darkfield microscope, can determine if yeast is present in the blood.

Symptoms

Symptoms of systemic yeast infections include fatigue, memory and concentration problems, bloating, digestive complaints, skin rashes and headaches.

Yeast infections are often due to the overuse of antibiotics. Even if you don't take antibiotics directly, all commercially raised animals receive antibiotics, which are passed to consumers via consumption of meat and dairy. Estrogen-like hormones are also added to animal feed which further aggravates this problem. High blood sugar increases yeast infections. High blood sugar can be caused by eating sugary foods and other carbohydrates (breads, bagels, donuts, pasta), diabetes, pregnancy, and excess estrogen. The estrogen connection is particularly interesting. Estrogen dominance is linked to every female issue we are discussing in this book. Not only are yeast infections, especially if chronic, *caused by* excess estrogen, the overgrowth of yeast, in turn, *causes* excess estrogen because the yeast organisms release estrogen-like by-products!

Natural Help For Yeast Infections

Hygiene can control yeast infections. Allowing air to circulate in the groin area is a good idea. Loose cotton clothing is preferable to tight man-made fabrics that do not breathe. Tampons and feminine products such as spray deodorants and fragrances may aggravate the condition. The simple act of wiping after urinating from front to back can cut down on the possibility of fecal contamination. Rinsing the vaginal area with water after intercourse can cut down on reinfection via a male sex partner.

Dietary change is needed to control and eliminate yeast infections. This involves the decreased consumption of all sugary and high simple carbohydrate foods, with an increase in healthy vegetables and flaxseed oil. All meat and dairy products must be free range, organic, and antibiotic free.

Douching with herbal combinations can help to get rid of vaginal yeast; using commercial preparations with fragrance, dyes, and preservatives may make it worse.

YEAST INFECTION DOUCHE RECIPE

In large douche bag with 2 quarts of lukewarm water, mix together:

> ½ teaspoon acidophilus powder (this has more active acidophilus
>   culture than yogurt)
> 2 teaspoons Dr. Bronner's Liquid Peppermint Soap
> ¼ teaspoon tea tree oil
> ½ teaspoon boric acid (optional—use only with stubborn cases)

Douche twice a day until symptoms have cleared. Then use as a preventive measure following the end of the period and after sex.

CYCLES OF LIFE

Men do not have visible symptoms, but can still carry yeast and bacterial infections. This means that they can keep reinfecting women. If your yeast infection is chronic, even after a change of diet and the use of herbal therapies, have your male sex partner evaluated.

For the recipe for **YEAST INFECTION PESSARY,** see page 82.

HERBS TO ELIMINATE YEAST INFECTIONS: A combination of herbs can be taken orally. These include herbs that contain berberine, such as goldenseal and barberry root, citrus seed extract, coptis, garlic, black walnut, quassia fruit, artemesia, thyme, oregano, tea tree and clove. (*Plantibiotic* from Nature's Answer contains all of these.) These herbs help to eliminate microorganisms including yeast and bacteria (*Gardnerella, Trichomonas*) responsible for bacterial vaginitis. It is a good idea to replenish the system with friendly bacteria by taking a probiotic. Probiotics are bacterial cultures of acidophilus, bifidus, and other bacteria that are beneficial to our bodies and also help to control candida by competing with them for space to grow. Organic, unflavored yogurt can be helpful in providing your body with active beneficial bacterial cultures, but it is more effective to use a commercially prepared probiotic product available in health food stores.

Premenstrual Syndrome (PMS)—Premenstrual Crazies

Premenstrual syndrome, usually referred to as PMS, is a term understood by most women, and the men who live with them! In fact, it is the most common disorder experienced by women during the menstrual years, with some estimates claiming that 90 percent of women are affected by it. However, there is a vast difference in the symptoms that individuals experience. Many woman have just a few mild symptoms, while others suffer severe discomfort which adversely effects their quality of life. Common symptoms include: water retention, weight gain, bloating, breast tenderness, fatigue, migraines and headaches, acne and other skin disruptions, depression, moodiness, irritability, carbohydrate and sweet cravings, insomnia, constipation. The bulk of these symptoms occur five to seven days before the period begins, although some woman begin to have symptoms shortly after ovulation, and so are spending half of each month in discomfort.

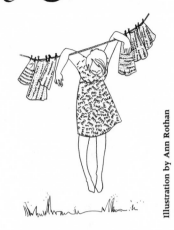

Illustration by Ann Rothan

NUTRITION FOR PMS: PMS is one health condition that even conventional medicine suggests has dietary causes. Some of the well known culprits include too much caffeine, sugar, artificial sweeteners, processed foods, and hydrogenated fats; lack of exercise; and a generally unhealthy lifestyle. Many women have experienced a marked decrease in the severity of PMS symptoms after adopting a healthy lifestyle, even if PMS was not the motivation. We often see this in natural healing—whenever a person makes the decision to eat an all natural, organic diet; begins to exercise daily; and practices stress reduction through meditation, prayer, yoga, biofeedback, or some other technique, the primary health problem is alleviated as well as other secondary annoyances. This lifestyle commitment helps to reverse the estrogen dominance that is another root cause of PMS. (See Estrogen Dominance, page 28.)

HERBS FOR PMS: Guy Abraham, M.D., was instrumental in classifying the symptoms of PMS into four main categories, and in establishing the role of nutrition in PMS.[6] The four categories are mentioned here, along with herbs that can be helpful:

PMS-A (anxiety)—mood swings, irritability, crying jags
   Herbs: **Black cohosh**, soy, flax oil, **chaste berry, Dong quai, St. John's wort**

PMS-H (hyperhydration)—bloating, weight gain, water retention, breast tenderness, constipation
   Herbs: Liver support and diuretic herbs like **dandelion, burdock, milk thistle,** corn silk, **cascara sagrada** for constipation

PMS-C (cravings)—many symptoms of hypoglycemia (low blood sugar) like fatigue, vertigo (dizziness), sweet cravings, bingeing, heart palpitations, headaches
   Herbs: Gymnena sylvestre, linden flower, hawthorne berries, **Siberian ginseng**

PMS-D (depression)—crying bouts, insomnia, confusion, depression
   Herbs: **St. John's wort, Dong quai,** valerian, **rose bud,** and **Siberian ginseng**

One of the best herbal formulas for PMS is a Chinese patent medicine that goes by the name of *Women's Eight Treasure Pills* or *Women's Precious Pills*. (See page 110.)

The Menstruating Years

Menstrual Pain

Once the period begins many women report almost immediate relief from most PMS symptoms. Bloating, breast tenderness, and headaches diminish. However, the symptoms may be replaced during the first few days of the menstrual flow by menstrual pain. As with many female health issues, menstrual pain can vary greatly from individual to individual, as well as in the same person from month to month. Menstrual pain may be no more than an awareness, or mild, intermittent cramping, or severe debilitating pain that requires complete bed rest. Natural healing is very effective for menstrual cramps. Massage, acupuncture, deep breathing, and yoga stretching can all bring relief.

> HERBS FOR MENSTRUAL PAIN: Crampbark, **corydalis (Yan Hou Su), Dong quai**, and **Jamaican dogwood.** Several of these herbs are combined in *Botanodyne* (www.naturesanswer.com). Essential oil can be rubbed directly over the uterus and on the lower back. (See menstrual pain formula, page 84). Use a castor oil pack for additional relief.

Cystic and Fibroid Conditions— Ovaries, Breasts, Endometriosis, Uterine Fibroids

During the many years that I have helped women overcome these health issues, I have found that whether cysts or fibroid growths are a problem in the ovaries, the breasts, or the uterus, the same basic treatments will help. Endometriosis will also often respond to the lifestyle changes and herbal protocols discussed in this section.

One of the most disturbing problems associated with these conditions is the fear generated by the suspicion that the pain, swelling, and palpable lumpy areas that can accompany any of these problems may be due to cancer. Be sure to visit your health care practitioner for a medical diagnosis to rule out cancer, and to confirm your condition. Conventional techniques including blood tests and sonograms are excellent tools that your doctor may use to correctly diagnose your problem.

ESTROGEN DOMINANCE
A Major Cause of Cystic and Fibroid Conditions

All of these conditions are caused by a multitude of factors—genetic, psychological, and physical. But they all have at least one cause in common: too much aggressive estrogen, especially if the ratio of estrogen to progesterone is out of balance, with estrogen dominating. There are many causes of estrogen dominance. In rare cases it can be caused by a genetic abnormality. However, it usually is influenced by lifestyle choices, which women *do* have control over. One of the main reasons women have too much estrogen is due to all the estrogens that are coming into their bodies from inorganic food and environmental toxins. These are called xenoestrogens.

Xenoestrogens—
A Common Cause of Estrogen Dominance

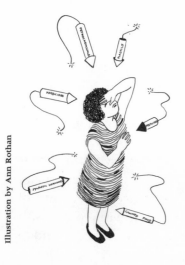

Illustration by Ann Rothan

Xenoestrogens are estrogen-like compounds that are highly toxic. They are found throughout the environment as by-products of pesticides, herbicides, and the synthetic hormones routinely fed to animals, which is stored in their fat and transferred to people who eat them. They also come from petrochemicals found in the coating inside canned food, and other plastics, even baby bottles! Once inside the body, xenoestrogens can be strong carcinogens, and may initiate cell growth associated with non-cancerous tumors such as uterine fibroids and fibrocystic breasts. They compete with more mild forms of estrogen for specific receptor cites, and play havoc with the "normal" mechanisms of the reproductive cycle.

Factors That Cause Estrogen Dominance

- Stress, especially if prolonged over time
- Food containing pesticides and herbicides (anything that is not organic)
- Hydrogenated fats found in margarine, baked goods, fried foods
- Poor diet—insufficient amounts of dark green leafy vegetables and organic fruits
- Sedentary lifestyle—not getting enough exercise
- Birth control pills
- Chronic yeast infections (Yeast releases estrogen-like compounds.)
- Toxic liver (The liver breaks down estrogen and cannot do so efficiently if it is overburdened.)
- Low progesterone levels due to stress (progesterone converts to stress hormones), low vitamin B-6, low magnesium levels, or low production of progesterone
- Sluggish bowels: fewer than one or two bowel movements per day (Excess estrogen and other toxins remains in the body too long and may be reabsorbed.)
- Sluggish circulation of body fluids—blood and lymph (Symptoms such as breast cysts or tender breasts associated with PMS are actually swollen lymph glands.)
- Low thyroid function—may be undiagnosed by conventional medicine

CYCLES OF LIFE

Self-Help Program to Decrease Estrogen Dominance

Since a multitude of factors contributes to the out-of-balance status that can lead to the development of cysts and fibroids and estrogen dominance, there is no one pill answer; not in the form of a synthetic drug or a natural herb. However, the good news is these conditions may be a wake-up call. To rid the body of these growths requires a dedication to a lifestyle that leads to overall health and wellness. It is best to work with a knowledgeable health care practitioner for individual guidance and monitoring. However, no one can actually make these lifestyle choices for anyone else—it is each woman for herself!

Following is a self-help program that you can use to balance many of the factors that cause estrogen dominance.

Detoxification

Following a full detoxification program (see page 18) is the first and possibly the most important step in decreasing estrogen dominance.

Stress Reduction

Scientific research has monitored stress indicators such as the release of specific hormones, blood oxygenation level and respiration and heart rate. You may want to consider seeing a psychologist or psychotherapist to help sort out emotional stress in your life. There are also specific self-help techniques that can be used to move the entire physiology, as well as the mind, into a more relaxed state. Yoga, meditation, and prayer are three of these techniques. Practicing yoga or tai chi for half an hour per day can help to decrease stress and regulate hormone function.

It is interesting to consider the mind/body connection in the development of endometriosis. This problem is most often seen in women who have never been pregnant. There is no confirmed physiological reason for this. Perhaps it is the body's own innate intelligence attempting to fulfill some kind of encoded mission!

Through deep meditation and positive self-talk perhaps we can program a new intelligence into our cells.

Mini De-Stress Break: Set aside a sacred time on a daily basis. Even a short amount of time is helpful. For instance, arrive at work five minutes early. Stay in your car. Turn the cell phone off. Have a copy of your Bible or any sacred book in the car. Breathe in deeply and exhale slowly three times. Read one short segment in the Bible. Then think about it for a few minutes. If you prefer, play a tape of relaxing music while you breathe deeply. Longer breaks are even better. They give the body a chance to truly unwind, which ultimately has the effect of lowering stress hormones and help balancing estrogen and progesterone.

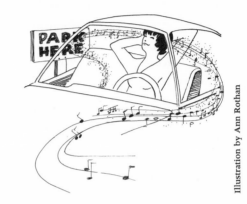

Illustration by Ann Rothan

De-Stressing Bath: Take a hot bath with 1 cup of baking soda, 1 cup of sea salt, and 10 drops of lavender oil for half an hour, three times per week. This especially helps draw toxins out through the skin if you are doing a detoxification program—also necessary to get rid of cysts and fibroids. Precede bath with dry skin brushing (see page 21).

HERBS TO HELP RELIEVE STRESS: **St. John's wort**, **kava kava**, valerian, hops

---

Decrease Exposure to Xenoestrogens

Become more conscious of xenoestrogens and avoid them as much as possible. This includes increased consumption of organic foods, dark green leafy vegetables (kale, swiss chard, collard greens) nutritious herbs (**green foods, sea vegetables**). Cut out all processed food and all food additives. Reduce consumption of animal products. Use small amounts of fish, meat, dairy, eggs, and other animal products that are free-range or organically raised. Include Omega-3 oils in the diet. Good sources of Omega-3s include flax seeds (2–3 tablespoons a day) and the herb, purslane (1 cup).

Use natural cleaning fluids in your home such as baking soda and vinegar. There are many naturally based cleaners in the health food store. Switch to shampoo and toothpaste that is naturally based. Get a water filter for your kitchen faucet and your shower. Hire an organic gardener to care for your lawn. Avoid "ChemGrass" or any similar company. In general, cut down on your exposure to toxins. Unfortunately, they are all around us and if you are not proactive in avoiding them, you are definitely being exposed.

Exercise daily

Find some form of movement you enjoy and do it at least half an hour every day. Yoga and tai chi can double as a stress reduction technique and exercise—what a bargain! Walking one mile daily or jumping on a small mini-trampoline are also excellent choices. Trampoline jumping has the added advantage of simulating a sluggish lymphatic system, one of the culprits in fibroid and cystic conditions. Trampoline jumping also gets rid of cellulite!

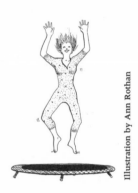

Illustration by Ann Rothan

Raising Progesterone Levels

In natural healing we prefer to address the cause of low progesterone levels through the use of diet, nutrients, and herbs rather than just taking synthetic progesterone. (Synthethic progesterone such as *Provera* does not have the same chemical structure as our body's own progesterone and can have severe side effects.)

NUTRITION FOR RAISING PROGESTERONE: One cause of low progesterone is a deficiency of vitamin B-6. Supplementing with this nutrient is recommended (250 mg/day). Food sources include Brewer's yeast, desiccated liver, soybeans, and blackstrap molasses. The hormone prolactin interferes with the function of the corpus luteum which produces progesterone. Low magnesium levels are associated with low progesterone and elevated prolactin. Supplement with magnesium. especially a highly absorbable form such as magnesium glycinate (1000 mg/day). Good food sources of magnesium are dark green leafy vegetables and almonds.

HERBS FOR RAISING PROGESTERONE: Chlorophyll, the green substance inside of plants, has a very similar chemistry as our own blood, except that chlorophyll contains magnesium instead of iron. Therefore **green foods**, **sea vegetables** and green vegetable juice are helpful. Herbs that are known to help increase Progesterone levels include **chaste berries** and **wild yam**. **Wild yam** is often used as an ingredient in progesterone cream, which is used topically on the skin to raise progesterone levels (see page 157).

Balancing Thyroid Function

Your thyroid gland may be underfunctioning, even though conventional medical tests don't pick this up. Visit a knowledgeable natural health care practitioner for further testing if you suspect this may be a problem for you. You can also try the following test yourself.

Temperature Test for Low Thyroid Function: Get a basal thermometer at any pharmacy. Get Styrofoam cups with lids and have them available in the bathroom. First thing in the morning, urinate into the cup. Put lid on tightly and insert thermometer into urine. Take reading and record on graph paper. Repeat every day for one or two months. If the average temperature of your morning urine is less than 97.8 degrees, you probably have an underactive thyroid even if your blood tests are within normal range.

If you find this temperature to be low and you have several of the following symptoms, your thyroid may be underfunctioning. Your body may be manufacturing enough thyroid hormone, but the ability to bind to and stimulate tissues may be impaired.

Symptoms of Underfunctioning Thyroid: Fatigue, depression, weight gain, sensitivity to cold, infertility, excessive menstrual flow, severe cramps, joint pain, migraines, dry skin, limp thin hair, cognitive problems, anemia, low sex drive are just a few of the forty-seven recognized clinical symptoms of low thyroid function.

NATURAL HELP FOR LOW THYROID: If low thyroid is due to an iodine deficiency, adding **sea vegetables**, especially **kelp**, to the diet will help. The yoga posture known as the "Shoulder Stand" followed by "The Fish" helps to exercise and stimulate the thyroid gland. Use a **castor oil** pack (see page 100), on the skin over the thyroid gland for 45 minutes three times a week. Repeat temperature test after three months. If there is no improvement, supplementation with *Synthroid* or *Armor-Thyroid* may be necessary and must be prescribed by a physician.

CHAPTER FOUR

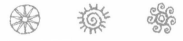

Fertility

Choosing our time to become parents is an important decision. Herbs have been used throughout human history to influence reproduction, both through natural birth control methods and through fertility enhancement.

NATURAL BIRTH CONTROL

Before starting a discussion about herbs that have been used as natural birth control, I need to strongly make the following point. *I do not recommend relying on the use of herbs or other natural methods of birth control, especially if you are at a point in life where pregnancy is definitely not an option.* Herbs may be useful for a married couple who would *prefer* not to conceive, or for someone who suffers drastic side effects from conventional birth control methods. Even in those situations, I have personally seen negative consequences after relying on herbs alone as a birth control method. These include unwanted pregnancies and severe infections after failed attempts of herb induced abortions. Please use the following information judiciously, or better yet, simply include it in your data bank of knowledge—without throwing away the condoms and diaphragms!

HERBS USED HISTORICALLY FOR CONTRACEPTION: **Wild yam** *(Dioscorea species)*, **wild carrot/Queen Ann's lace** *(Daucus carota)*, **burning bush (Dictamnus albas), castor oil, rue** *(Ruta graveolens)*

Other Natural Contraception Methods

Besides herbal remedies, other forms of natural contraception are available. These include the *fern test*, the *mucus test*, and the *rhythm method*. All of these methods help a woman to determine when she is most likely to be fertile. This information can be used both to decrease or increase the possibility of becoming pregnant.

Fern Test

It is amazing to find the intricate interrelationships between the plant, animal, and mineral kingdoms. The body's fluids are cyclic in nature, as are our hormones. One amazing phenomena, which was discovered by science in the 1940s yet is still not widely known by mainstream medicine, is the fact that our body fluids, particularly saliva, will dry in different crystalline patterns according to our hormone levels—this relates to fertility status. Early in the menstrual cycle, before the maturation of the egg, while the woman is not fertile, the saliva will dry into dots. The pattern will change to straight lines just before and during ovulation. Right after ovulation a branched fern-like pattern will emerge in the dried saliva!

This test is accomplished with the use of a tiny, inexpensive microscope. A women touches her tongue to the lens of the microscope and allows the saliva to dry. She then views the patterns formed in the dry saliva. After several months of use, the time of fertility can be predicted with some degree of accuracy. This empowers a woman with self-care information that can be useful to avoid or enhance the chances of conception (see Resources, on page 185, for fern test equipment).

Mucus Test

You can check your own cervical mucus by inserting a finger vaginally and observing the color, consistency, and "stickiness" of the mucus. Each woman will vary as to what is normal; however, if practiced consistently, knowledge about your cycle will increase. You should notice and record patterns of change that occur during the month. At the time of fertility you will probably see that the mucus changes in consistency and becomes less tacky. Instead, it will become more stringy and slippery with a consistency similar to raw egg white. It will often form a thin string between two fingers as they are pulled apart. Intercourse should be avoided for a few days before the expected change of the mucus to the stringy form if you wish to avoid pregnancy.

Rhythm Method

The rhythm method has been used for many years by people who want to time the arrival of children but who have religious or philosophical beliefs that do not include the use of contraceptives. The rhythm method uses simple calculation (see pages 38–39) to plot the expected time of ovulation. Intercourse is then avoided for a few days before and during ovulation. A new and improved version of the rhythm method is called the *Sympto-Thermal Method*; it uses a combination of timing and symptoms—such as the change in mucus described above—to determine fertility, and is taught by the Couple-Couple League (see Resources, page 185).

CYCLES OF LIFE

FERTILITY ENHANCEMENT

Conceiving a child is not as easy as you might expect. At least 25 percent of women report having trouble conceiving.[7] This high rate of infertility is due to several factors. Many modern women are starting families at a later age than in the past due to education, careers, and a tendency to marry later in life. Plus, nutritional deficiencies and environmental toxicity increase the disruption of normal hormonal function. If a woman has been living on the standard american diet based heavily on over processed, devitalized products, baked goods, fried foods, antibiotic and hormone filled meats, pesticide and herbicide laden produce, she is most likely deficient in several nutrients needed for optimum health, as well as fertility. She is also likely to have high levels of xenobiotics and xenoestrogens, toxic substances that play havoc with our hormonal balance. This holds true for men as well as women, since sperm count and activity are also affected. If you are having trouble conceiving, be sure to have a complete workup by a competent fertility specialist to rule out blockages and other obvious physical problems. Once these are ruled out, changes in diet and lifestyle, along with the use of specific herbs, and several drug free, non-invasive methods can improve your chances of conception.

Ovulation Detection Methods

The first step you should take to increase your chances of conceiving is to chart your ovulation, so that you will know when you are most fertile.

Calculating Ovulation

To find out when you are most likely to ovulate, keep track of how many days are between the first day of one period and the first day of the next period. Do this for several months. Ovulation occurs fourteen days before the next menstrual cycle begins. After several menstrual cycles are calendared, subtract fourteen days from the longest cycle and fourteen days from the shortest cycle. For example, if you have 29-, 31-, and 30-day cycles, the longest cycle is 31 − 14 = 17; the shortest cycle is 29 − 14 = 15. You will most likely ovulate between day fifteen and day seventeen on your average cycle. Your efforts at conception should be focused around these dates.

Basal Body Temperature Mapping (BBT)

To calculate your BBT, you will need a pen, graph paper, and a basal thermometer (available in any drug store). First, prepare a chart by writing the numbers 1 through 31 in a vertical column down the side of the graph paper. These correspond to the dates of the month. Then, across the top, write values for temperature. Start with 95 and increase by .2 for each line—95, 95.2, 95.4, and so on, until you reach 100. Most basal thermometers have a chart included so you don't have to make your own. Take your temperature each morning after a good night's sleep, while still lying in bed, before you even sit up. The materials needed should be placed in reach of the bed. After you have the reading, find the point on the graph that most closely matches the reading and record it by placing a dot in that spot. The BBT should be recorded every day until the next menstrual period.

Chart Interpretation: The first phase of the menstrual cycle generally has only slight temperature fluctuations. Upon ovulation, there may or may not be a dip in temperature, but there should always be a 1.0- to 1.5-degree (F) rise in temperature in the luteal phase (days 18 to 21). This elevation will continue until one to two days before the next period. If the temperature rise does not last ten to twelve days, you may be experiencing a short luteal phase. This rise in temperature occurs in response to increased progesterone secreted by the corpus luteum. After a general pattern is seen, intercourse should be planned two days prior to anticipated ovulation, at an interval of every forty-eight hours. If you are supplementing with progesterone, be aware that it may falsely raise the temperatures and invalidate BBT results. A flat temperature chart is indicative of a cycle where no ovulation has occurred. Temperatures that remain elevated may indicate pregnancy.

Cervical Mucus Monitoring

Changes that occur to the cervical mucus during the menstrual cycle can often help determine fertility. Insert finger intravaginally each day, and note and chart changes in mucus for several months. This can act as an invaluable self-assessment tool. After a menstrual period has ended, the vagina is usually dry with little to no mucus. Just before ovulation the mucus production increases in response to increasing levels of estrogen. This special mucus is called *ovulation mucus*. It is a necessary component for successful fertilization. Ovulation mucus has some outstanding characteristics. It forms a corridor pattern within the vagina, stretching from the opening to the *os*, or mouth of the uterus. This corridor guides sperm to the egg. The strings of this corridor mucus have a frequency pattern within the same range as the frequency patterns of the tails of sperm cells. This mucus is also high in glucose and other nutrients that nourish sperm cells and keep them alive for up to five days, increasing chances of fertilization. It usually becomes creamy, wet, and whitish in color. Intercourse should be initiated when these mucus changes are noted, and repeated every forty-eight hours during this phase. Upon ovulation, the mucus changes again. It becomes clear, thin, and stretchy. Its appearance is similar to that of an egg white. Intercourse should continue during this time.

The consistency of cervical mucus can be affected by intercourse, infection, showering, bathing, douching, recent birth control pill use, and lower levels of estrogen.

Fern Test

See pages 36–37.

Fertility

Home Ovulation Detection Kits

These kits are now widely available in drugstores. They are based on the measurement of LH that occurs just prior to ovulation. Although there is no guarantee, ovulation should occur within 12 to 16 hours after the test is positive.

If you have decided to try natural remedies to increase your chances of conception, there are several herbs that you can consider.

HERBS TO ENHANCE FERTILITY:

Chaste Tree (*Vitex agnus-castus*)—helps to balance progesterone levels which are often too low in the second half of an infertile woman's cycle.

Black Cohosh (*Cimicifuga racemosa*)—helps balance estrogen; can restart periods.

Damiana (*Turnera aphrodisiaca*)—used as an aphrodisiac for both men and women, increases sexual desire.

Ho Shou Wu—used in China for centuries as a longevity tonic and fertility enhancement.

False Unicorn Root—helps to balance uterine function, most renowned fertility herb.

Red Raspberry—nutritious balancing herb for women; helps with infertility and is safe to use throughout pregnancy.

Other Natural Methods to Increase Fertility

Besides the use of herbs and nutrients, the energy techniques of ritual and creative visualization can yield remarkable results in aiding fertility. Many couples have claimed that these methods seemed to really "turn the tide" in their quest to establish a family.

CYCLES OF LIFE

Adoption

When women visit me specifically for help with fertility I always ask them if they have considered adoption. The adoption process can be long, involved, and arduous, and usually requires about two years. I encourage couples to begin the process because the end result of parenthood is assured, and because there is a miraculous occurrence which I, and many other fertility specialists have witnessed—pregnancy often occurs shortly after adoption proceedings have been initiated. Perhaps the release of stress helps to balance the hormones sufficiently to allow pregnancy to occur. If it does happen, the couple can cancel the adoption proceedings. If pregnancy does not occur, they still are moving towards parenthood. Many couples have had a biological child and completed the adoption process anyway, having a whole family all at once. This has worked out quite well especially with couples who are older when they begin the child bearing phase of life.

Creating Space

While taking a history of a woman who is experiencing difficulty conceiving, she will often share details with me about her hectic lifestyle. Many of these women are professionals with demanding career schedules, after work activities, and household responsibilities. I ask, "How do you think you will have time for a baby?" I am often greeted with an aghast expression after such a comment. However, it is an important consideration. The energy field that surrounds us—call it aura, bioelectric energy, chi, life force—has an innate intelligence. It "knows" our challenges, stresses, and limits; perhaps better than our ego-based mind. If a woman's schedule is already stressed to the breaking point, that may be a factor that scares off a potential pregnancy. I counsel would-be mothers to begin to create sacred space in their life. This may mean cutting back work hours, giving up some civic duties, and scaling down social commitments. Take serious time to sit home, to nest, to imagine caring for a baby. Put out the mental psychic energy to the universe that you *do* have the time, space, love, and patience needed for parenthood. Herbs can be used as a ritual during this time. Burn sage in an abalone shell. Brush the sage smoke over yourself with a feather that you find during a walk in the woods. While you brush the smoke call out loud to your own grandmothers, and plead your case. State your intention to bring a child into the world. Be specific about why this is important to you. Feel the internal excitement of your desire!

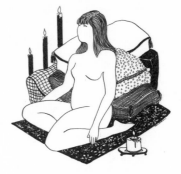

Illustration by Ann Rothan

Visualization Aids

Here is an effective visualization aid that you can try. Get a large piece of oaktag. Cut out pictures from magazines to create a collage. Design it so it represents what you hope to create in your life. Fill the blank sheet with pictures of pregnant women, babies, families walking down the street with a stroller, and whatever else conjures a picture of the scene you would like to see in your own life. Place the completed collage near your bed. Allow yourself to look at it through half-closed eyes as you drift off to sleep, and as soon as you awaken. After looking at the images, create a movie in your mind before you go to sleep. Remember, you are the star, the producer, and the director. Allow your vision to be the apex of the best, happiest, healthiest scene you can imagine. After a week or two of doing this exercise you may start to have actual dreams about the happy family you have. In a mystical way, your body may be prompted to bring this vision into reality. Perhaps it helps to balance hormones, perhaps it opens the doors to new souls who wish to incarnate, perhaps we'll never know how it works. However, if often does the trick!

CHAPTER FIVE

Pregnancy

DURING PREGNANCY

Pregnancy is one of the most joyous, yet difficult cycles of life. The body changes on so many levels. Hormones fluctuate, the body shape changes, causing stretching and pulling on bones, muscles, tendons, and skin. Psychological changes also take place.

Nutrition During Pregnancy

Placing extra attention on nutrition both for you and the growing fetus is paramount during this time. Include **sea vegetables**, **green drinks**, **nettle**, lots of organic fruits and vegetables, organic yogurt if dairy is tolerated, free-range meats and poultry, and omega-3 oils. Studies have shown that the essential fatty acid DHA can have beneficial neurological effects on newborns if their mother had sufficient amounts during pregnancy.[8] DHA is part of the DHA-EPA complex found in fatty fish such as salmon and mackerel. Vegetarian sources include red and brown algae (sea vegetables) and nutritional supplement capsules. If nausea is a

45

problem, eat very small amounts of healthy foods, even just a spoonful at a time, throughout the day instead of large meals. Increase consumption of bioflavonoids found in fruits, especially berries like bilberries, blueberries, cranberries and raspberries.

Herbs During Pregnancy

Many modern women are reticent to use herbs during pregnancy, fearing it may harm the fetus. Actually, herbs have been used to complement and ease the discomforts of pregnancy in every civilization throughout history. However, since many chemical constituents in herbs are capable of passing through the placenta, it is better to play it safe. *Don't use* any herb *(or pharmaceutical drug for that matter) without checking reliable sources to determine its safety for use during pregnancy.* Since there are so many metabolic changes that occur, the reaction that herbs have in your body may be different during pregnancy. Extra caution should be exercised during the first trimester of early pregnancy to avoid anything that can cause uterine contraction and initiate miscarriage. Even commonly used herbs such as goldenseal should not be used during early pregnancy.

Overall Support—**Red raspberry** leaf tea or tincture can be used safely throughout pregnancy. It supports the body and mind of the expectant mother with additional nutrients such as calcium, and has a gentle calming effect.

Morning Sickness/Nausea—**Wild yam** cream used on the stomach may help nausea. **Ginger** is extremely helpful. Ginger tea is available in tea bags at health food stores. Or you can make your own ginger tea, with peppermint and cinnamon for added relief.

GINGER TEA

2 Tbs sliced or grated fresh ginger root
1 fresh spring (about 1 inch) peppermint, or 1 tsp dried leaves
1 cinnamon stick or ⅛ tsp cinnamon powder

Steep above ingredients in one quart boiled water for 10 minutes. Make a large batch and drink hot, cold, or at room temperature.

Pregnancy

Keep ginger tea at your bedside along with small rice cakes to consume first thing in the morning to allay nausea. If you don't like the taste of ginger, it is available as capsules or tablets. The Chinese patent medicine *Pill Curing Formula* is also very helpful for morning sickness.

Constipation—Use fiber and bulking agents like psyllium seeds and flax seeds. Increase fruit consumption. Dandelion can also be helpful. Avoid aggressive laxatives such as senna. Cascara should be used in very small amounts only if bulking agents don't help.

Colds/Flus—Echinacea and vitamin C can help. Drink echinacea tea with lemon, honey, and half a clove of garlic, up to six cups a day. Use eucalyptus as an inhalant: boil eucalyptus leaves in water, cover your head with a towel, and inhale the steam.

Varicose Veins are considered an unsightly cosmetic problem; however, they can be more problematic than that, and may increase the risk of developing leg ulcers. Varicose veins may occur in the outer vaginal lips or the legs during the stresses of pregnancy. Increasing bioflavonoid consumption can help. Berries and fruits are high in bioflavonoids. *Joint Phytonutrition* (see www.naturesanswer.com) is a very concentrated source of bioflavonoids. External compresses of **horse chestnut** and **oatmeal** have a soothing astringent effect, and can be applied during pregnancy.

Stretch Marks can be effectively avoided by using a combination of vitamin E oil, almond oil, and aloe vera. Adding cocoa butter gives the mixture a pleasing aroma and adds to the emollient quality. Rub it on the entire abdomen area daily, as well as on the breasts, and any other area of skin that seems to be stretching during pregnancy. Take 2 to 3 tablespoons of flax oil a day and supplement with vitamin E (mixed tocopherols, 400 IU/day).

Anxiety is common in pregnant women. Hormone swings, shifting body image, worry about the change in lifestyle that is imminent with the birth of a new baby all add up to increased anxiety. Daily slow stretching and deep breathing along with gentle yoga

47

postures and relaxing music are useful. Herbal tea made from **chamomile** flowers can be used, especially after the first trimester, and is relaxing at bedtime. **Oatstraw** is safe during pregnancy and is high in minerals such as calcium and magnesium which soothes the nerves.

Music and Healing Sounds During Pregnancy

Music can be safely used as a stress reduction tool during pregnancy. Sound waves easily travel through air and water. Your baby can feel vibrations of sounds, your voice, and even your emotions. Taking the time to send healing tones into your body during pregnancy can help to precipitate an easy birth experience.

When I was pregnant with my first child, I was living on a farm in Arizona. A man from West Virginia lived next door, he was a dulcimer maker. The dulcimer is a string instrument of American origin that sits on the players lap. He made me a dulcimer out of special wood, and I chose a sacred turquoise stone that he carved into the handle. The instrument fit right up against by stomach when I was sitting. Every day, during my pregnancy, I played special songs to my unborn son, who was soothed by the instrument even after he was born.

LABOR
Birth Ecstasies

Labor was considered an initiation process in cultures throughout the ages. In the 1950s, in the United States, it became fashionable to use strong drugs to put the expectant mother "out," so that she could avoid the pain of childbirth. Women were strapped down to the delivery table on their backs with their feet up in stirrups. This made the birth process much more difficult. Hospital rules and regulations forbade the presence of fathers or midwives in the delivery room. In most cultures, women give birth in a semi-sitting position. Gravity and the mother's ability to actively push at the proper time aids the birthing process. With an unconscious mother in a supine position it was often necessary for physicians to resort to forceps and other artificial interventions. This process has many potential side effects including an increased incidence of postpartum blues. Believe it or not, many indigenous cultures have no word in their language for postpartum blues!

In the 1960s and 1970s, there was a movement initiated by women who did not want to be subjected to this kind of birth process. They wanted to fully experience the initiation of going through labor. Unfortunately, at that time there was no choice for these women within a hospital setting. The only way to escape the standard procedure was to opt for a home delivery.

From 1973 to 1977, I assisted women in home deliveries as a lay midwife. It was an amazing experience to share with my naturally oriented sisters. I had the good fortune to apprentice with shaman healers in Mexico, where the midwife tradition had remained part of the culture for thousands of years. I learned from these beautiful traditional healers how chanting, drumming, prayer, oils, and herbs can be used during labor to ease the process for the mother and to gently welcome the precious newborn into the world. How totally different from the hospital delivery room!

By the end of the twentieth century conventional obstetricians had once again embraced a more natural birth experience. Today midwives have become more popular and many modern hospitals now have birthing centers where fathers and friends can participate in a natural experience, while hospital facilities are readily available if needed. This is truly a blending of the best of both worlds!

Herbs to Ease Labor

The herbs discussed in this section should not be used without the supervision of a knowledgeable midwife, herbalist, or health care practitioner. Most can increase the strength and smoothness of contractions, but some have properties similar to the drug Pitocin (but with fewer side effects), and are called oxytocic. This means they help to facilitate child birth by stimulating uterine contractions.

- **Red raspberry** can be used throughout pregnancy.
- **Sea vegetables** and **green foods** are nutritive tonics.

- **Blue cohosh** can be taken close to the time of birth. About one week before expected delivery, drink 1 cup of tea or 10 drops of tincture/extract per day.
- **Castor oil** has been scientifically documented to shorten delivery time.[9] Take a half-teaspoon a day, for a few days prior as well as during labor.
- **Black cohosh** strengthens contractions if true labor has started, but stops false labor known as Braxton-Hicks contractions.
- **Nettle, burdock,** and **motherwort** can be combined and used as a tea to sip during labor.
- **Kava kava** and **Jamaican dogwood** help mood elevation and pain. Indigenous women, who live in areas where these herbs grow, rely on them for relief of labor pains. They specifically help decrease lower back pain and spasm experienced during labor.

Herbal and Oil Compresses

Apply the following compress to the perineum for a few days prior to labor. Continue during labor, but use in between contractions for the comfort of the mother.

PERINEAL COMPRESS

Equal parts sesame oil and almond oil
1 tsp liquid vitamin E (or open one capsule)
A few drops lavender oil

Soak a clean washcloth in warm water. Ring it out. Place on perineum. Massage the area with the oil mixture. Midwives will gently stretch the area with a gloved finger and the oil mixture. Repeat frequently (3 to 4 times a day) before labor and once an hour during labor.

This treatment can often entirely avoid the need for episiotomy (cutting the perineum) during delivery.

POSTPARTUM

The period of time following the birth of a baby is very joyous, but can be quite stressful as well. Many women are overwhelmed with the new responsibility of caring for a newborn twenty-four hours a day. In indigenous societies the social structure usually includes specific rituals and care for the new mother. She is often surrounded by women who bathe and massage her while the infant is cared for. Even in the West, it is common for friends and family to chip in and take over household chores and food preparation as well as care for the new mother and infant. Herbs can be helpful for some of the specific health care issues often experienced after labor and delivery.

Herbs for Postpartum Issues

Afterbirth pains occur as the uterus begins to contract and return to its prepregnancy size and shape. It is often worse with second and third births. **Kava kava**, hops, **Jamaican dogwood**, and **corydalis (Yan Hou Su)** are extremely helpful. Apply a **castor oil** or **ginger** compress to uterine area and use the postpartum essential oil rub formula described on page 84.

Postpartum Depression, AKA Baby Blues, often starts when the mother's milk comes in, usually on the third day after birth. Until then, colostrum is exuded from the breast. This substance is rich in nutrients and immune stimulants that help the baby adjust to her new environment and avoid infection. On the third day milk will start to come in, often along with tears and feelings of melancholy. This mild depression is referred to as "baby blues" and is quite common. It is possible that the hormonal rush that causes letting down of milk also initiates the letting down of tears. Allow yourself to have these feelings without guilt or worry. **Rosebud** and **chamomile** tea is an appropriate soothing herb combination

51

for this time, along with an aromatherapy bath with ten drops of lavender oil, which can help lift the spirits. If the depression does not lift after a few days or becomes too intense to bear, consult with your health care practitioner.

Hemorrhoids—Hemorrhoids are aggravated by the pressure of the baby's head on the perineal area during labor, and can be painful for the first week or two after labor. Take a sitz bath with lavender essential oils, or prepare one of the following compresses:

HEMORRHOID SOOTHERS

1 potato
4 pieces okra
1 tsp oatmeal
1 Tbs aloe vera gel

Grate the potato. Cook the okra in a small amount of water and smash or pound into a paste. Add the oatmeal and Aloe Vera. Mix all ingredients together, and apply to hemorrhoid area. Cover with gauze.

½ cup milk of magnesia
4 cubes ice

Pour milk of magnesia onto the ice in a bowl. Allow the ice to melt completely. Soak a washcloth in the liquid, and apply to hemorrhoid area.

NURSING
Breastfeeding Bliss

The time spent nursing a newborn provides special bonding for mother and child. Nursing is now recognized by mainstream medicine to be the preferred form of nutrition for an infant, and mothers are encouraged to nurse if at all possible. The first order of importance in establishing a healthy milk flow is to have a quiet restful environment in which to nurse. The more a baby nurses, the more milk flow is stimulated.

Nutrition for Nursing

Proper nutrition is essential for milk production. Protein, vitamins, minerals, and essential fatty acids must be consumed in adequate amounts. **Oats, sea vegetables,** and **green foods** can help provide the extra nutrients needed at this cycle of life. This is a time to pay particular attention to organic food sources since harmful pesticides and herbicides can pass through the milk.

Herbs to Aid Nursing

Herbs taken by nursing mothers can often pass into her milk and effect the baby. This can have a good effect—mother and child both feeling mellow after some chamomile tea; or a negative one—baby breaks out in diaper rash after mother has eaten a lot of garlic!

Galactagogues are herbs that have been used traditionally to increase the flow of milk. These should be started in small amounts (1 cup of tea or 10 drops of tincture a day). They can then be increased once it is determined that no ill effects are experienced by mother or baby. Increasing fluids is very important. Any mild flavored, non-medicinal herb tea can be used as part of the daily fluid intake, but be sure to include at least two quarts of plain, filtered water. The following herbs are among those that have been used as galactagouges: blessed thistle, **chaste berry**, fennel seed, dill, **black cohosh, fenugreek**, **milk thistle, nettle,** hops.

Fenugreek may make baby's urine have a maple-syrup aroma. In rare cases this may lead to a misdiagnosis of maple syrup urine disease in an infant. Hops are very popular for inducing milk production. Hops are used to make beer, an old favorite of nursing mothers. Drinking some beer before nursing can help induce a tranquil state, allowing milk to flow more freely. A study in the medical journal *Lancet* (April 29, 2000), reports that Vitamin B-6 concentrations increase after drinking beer. Vitamin B-6 is essential for all areas of female wellness.

Breast Engorgement or milk fever occurs when milk ducts become blocked. This can lead to areas of the breast becoming hot, red, and sometimes hard or swollen. If left untreated this condition may lead to a whole body infection. However, in most cases, you can help to avoid or treat this problem through the application of hot compresses to the reddened area, expressing milk manually, and/or allowing the baby to nurse. Participating in La Leche League meetings (see www.lalecheleague.org) can arm a new mother with information on how to handle such an occurrence. It is wise to attend La Leche League meetings for three to four months before the baby's birth.

BREAST COMPRESS

3 Tbs dried nettle leaf or 30 drops nettle tincture
1 Tbs grated ginger root
2 Tbs lavender flower tops or 5 drops lavender essential oil
1 tsp ground fenugreek seeds
1 quart water

Mix all ingredients together. Heat, but do not boil. Allow to cool just enough to be able to touch. Soak a clean wash cloth in the solution. Cover the entire breast, focusing on the affected area. Repeat several times until you notice a softening of the hardened area.

and/or

4–6 cabbage leaves

Steam cabbage leaves until soft. Allow to cool to body temperature, then wrap around breast for 20 to 30 minutes.

Sore or cracked nipples are more common if you don't prepare in advance by rubbing nipples daily during pregnancy with a terry cloth towel to toughen them. If sore or cracked nipples becomes a problem for you, use vitamin E, avocado oil, or almond oil on the nipples for a soothing effect.

BABY FORMULA

Here is a good recipe for natural baby formula if you cannot, or do not, wish to nurse, or for when your baby reaches weaning age. Many babies with severe allergies, colic, indigestion, diaper rash, and other problems thrive on this formula recipe.

> 8 oz. fresh or powdered goat milk, or organic cow milk
> 1 tsp flax oil
> 250 mg taurine
> ½ tsp acidophilus
> ¼ cc (for under 2 months old, 1 cc for older babies) liquid
>   children's multi-vitamins (available at health food stores)

Mix all ingredients. Pour in baby's bottle and warm bottle to body temperature by placing in warm water. DO NOT MICROWAVE!

CHAPTER SIX

Joys of Sex

Orgasmic Knowings

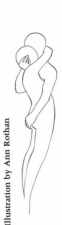

Illustration by Ann Rothan

Sex is a human experience that has influenced the course of history of entire civilizations, as well as being a formative force in the life of individuals. Humans are one of the only species that use sex for recreation, not only procreation. (Dolphins are also documented to engage in bisexual activity regularly, not only during fertile seasons.) Sexual activity is steeped in spirituality and mysticism. The schizophrenic nature of humankind's struggle with the powerful sexual force can be seen by the attempt to both deify and repress it. Opposing views on sexuality have come in and out of favor in various societies throughout the ages. The voluptuous erotic sculptures that adorn the ancient Hindu temples of India are transcendent and reflect the divine bliss experienced at the instant of orgasm. Other religious teachings take great pains to cover all parts of the body with non-erotic apparel in an attempt to sublimate the sexual nature.

Civilizations throughout the ages use sexuality as a conduit to transcend usual life experiences. The *Kama Sutra* is an ancient Hindu text that describes sexual positions in detail. Wilhelm Reich, an associate of Sigmund Freud, describes the energy released during orgasm as orgone energy, which, if used wisely, can decrease or reverse the aging process. Tantric yoga involves the use of the exchange of male and female energy to experience life as an androgynous full spectrum of reality—male and female learn sexual techniques to share life force energy. Wicca (a nature-based religion) uses sexual ritual to influence the forces of nature. There is a continuum of female sexual expression that can be represented by the pure virginal essence of the Mother Mary and the harlot image of Mary Magdalene. Women are free to choose to incorporate into their own self expression either or both images that these women represent. Perhaps the middle path is the road most traveled, with different phases being expressed at different times.

SEX AFTER MENOPAUSE

Of all the complaints and fears that women express about the effects of menopause the possibility of the loss of sexuality is most pervasive. However, in a recent study of 436 women, "little difference was found between age-matched subgroups of pre- and postmenopausal women in frequency of sexual behavior and attitudes towards their sexual relationships ."[10] Outcomes indicated that while frequency of sexual encounters decreased somewhat with age, enjoyment and satisfaction associated with sex was not related to age. In a very real sense, the old adage, "if you don't use it, you lose it" applies to sexual function. Women who continue to experience sexual stimulation, either with a partner or via masturbation exhibit less thinning and drying of the vagina after menopause.[11]

LOW LIBIDO

Woman of any age may experience a lessening of libido. This is often due to health conditions that lead to fatigue, stress, unhappy emotional relationships, and poor nutrition. There are also times when a woman may choose to purposely lessen her sexual focus and activity, such as while pursuing a time of internal self reflection and growth.

Techniques to Enhance Sexuality

Diet

The same diet that is used to detoxify the body and control excess aggressive estrogen will also balance hormone function, which leads to better sexual health. Certain foods are believed to increase sexuality. These include **oats**, **sea vegetables, green foods,** and shellfish, especially oysters.

Visualization

Using the mind to focus on erotic images can enhance the production of sex hormones. This can be a personal mind's eye movie created by the individual, or it can be through the use of videos, photos, or other visual stimulation.

Exercise

Regular exercise is paramount for increased sexual activity. Exercise tones, strengthens, and increases endurance. Both the psychological effects of having a positive self image and the physical effects of balanced hormone production and endorphin (feel-good chemicals) release that accompanies regular exercise helps out with sexual fitness. The sex act is good exercise in itself! It increases intracellular oxygenation, releases endorphins, slightly lowers bad cholesterol, increases estrogen production in women (especially in menopause), increases testosterone in both men and women, regulates menstrual cycles, increases the production of adrenal hormones, and burns calories and fat.

The Kegel Exercise is an exercise that is particularly effective at enhancing the sexual experience. This movement strengthens the muscles surrounding the vagina and the pubococcygeus (PC) muscle. It also has the benefit of avoiding or curing the problem of weak bladder control. The Kegel exercise is beneficial to both men and women. Exercising the PC muscle increases local blood and nutrient supplies, tones and increases elasticity and power, and can lead to enhanced sexual sensitivity and more intense orgasms; quite a lot of benefit from an exercise that can be done discreetly anywhere, anytime.

KEGEL EXERCISE

While urinating, attempt to stop the stream of fluid. Hold for a few seconds then release again. Do this several times. Continue to practice during every urination until you know how to isolate the PC muscle.

Incorporate the exercise into your daily life—not only while urinating. Squeeze the muscle and hold for two seconds, then release. Repeat five times. Do this two or three times a day. As you become comfortable increase the time you hold, and add repetitions. More advanced practice includes clamping the anal sphincter and adding in a bearing down movement, all without contracting the buttocks.

To aid in remembering to do the Kegel, you can coordinate it along with other daily life activities such as brushing your teeth. The time spent commuting to work is ideal—what better way is there to stay stress free in a traffic jam than to allow your mind to enjoy a sexual fantasy while you Kegel?

Joys of Sex

Herbs to Enhance the Joy of Sex

Womankind (and mankind too) has experimented with various plant substances throughout history in an endless search for useful aphrodisiacs. Many folklore tales of sexual potency are linked to herbs. Although some of these stories are probably just wishful thinking, there are some herbs that have stood the test of time in their ability to stimulate and sustain sexuality, either during a particular love making session or over a lifespan into advanced age.

PREPARE A POTENT "LOVE POTION"

Red raspberry extract
Red clover extract
Siberian ginseng extract
Ginger extract
Oat extract
Damiana extract
Fenugreek extract
Kava kava extract

These are some of the herbs that enhance female sexuality. Combine 20 drops of each extract in ½ cup warm water. Add ½ ounce of Amaretto or some other flavored liquor. Relax and enjoy!

Deer Antler, although not *technically* an herb, has been prized in Chinese medicine for centuries as a sexual stimulant. The expression "horny" may be linked to this fact. It is considered one of the strongest yang tonics. This animal-based product is harvested without harm to the animals, since they shed their antlers naturally. Scientific studies show that deer antler is useful for anemia. It can increase both the number of red blood cells as well as the amount of hemoglobin in red blood cells. In women, deer antler increases the strength of contraction and tone of the uterus. It has an adaptogenic effect and increases overall strength and endurance and

61

decreases fatigue, as supported by tests done on athletes. Current research is linking the use of deer antler, as well as the velvet that is scraped off, to many health enhancing effects including cartilage growth and repair, increase of IGF-1 (an indicator of the amount of human growth hormone, which tends to decrease with age), blood pressure and cholesterol balancing, enhanced immune function, and a decrease in stress related illness.

Panax Ginseng is recognized for thousands of years as a powerful tonic, which gives the user the strength and power of youth. Often called Chinese ginseng, this root resembles the human form in shape and is a powerful sexual tonic as well as an overall adaptogen.

Maca (Lepidium meyenii), also called Peruvian ginseng although it is unrelated to ginseng, is part of the cruciferous vegetable family like cabbage, kale, and broccoli. It grows in the Andes Mountains. The part of the plant used is the tuberous root structure. It is high in essential fatty acids; minerals (phosphorus, calcium, magnesium, zinc); vitamins B, C and E; various phytosterols; and other nutritional factors known for their importance to sexual function. When specific maca compounds, *macamides* and *macaenes*, were given to laboratory animals in controlled trials, the animals showed a significant increase in sexual function (*Urology*, April 2000). History reports that Incan warriors used maca before battle to increase strength and endurance. It has been used throughout recorded history up to the present day by both men and women as an aphrodisiac.

Muira Puama (Ptychopetalum olacoides), known as "warrior wood" and "potency wood," is used by the people of the northern Amazon area in Brazil for many health issues. It is considered a tonic for the neuromuscular system, and helps with joint pain, menstrual cramps, PMS symptoms, and mental disturbances. The entire plant is used in medicinal preparations, and contains sterols, including beta-sitosterol, which may account for its activity as a sexual stimulant. Muira Puama is listed in the *British Herbal Pharmacopoeia* and is recommended for the treatment of impotence. In Brazil, it is used by both men and women to increase libido and sexual performance. Studies in France have verified its usefulness for men for both libido and impotence.

Yohimbe (Pausinystalia yohimbe) is derived from bark stripped from a tall evergreen West African tree. In its native land Yohimbe may be made into a tea, smoked, or processed into a powder and sniffed. In the western world, yohimbine, the primary active constituent of yohimbe, is actually a prescription drug—*yohimbine hydrochloride*—used for erectile dysfunction in men. Yohimbe increases testosterone blood levels in both men and women, causing enhanced sex drive. It also stimulates circulation to the genitals. This is especially helpful for men with decreased penile circulation; it may also offset vaginal atrophy in women. Dosage is important with this herb. Stick to the label directions on the product you are using. Do not use if you have kidney or liver disease, high blood pressure, or heart arrhythmias. Possible side effects include anxiety, increased blood pressure, and facial hair growth in women. The *Journal of Urology* (February 1998) reported that these side effects are infrequent and reversible. It is interesting to note that some people who experience these effects with the herbal extract have no problem taking the prescription drug!

Essential Oils and Lubricants

Essential oils can enhance the sexual experience in several ways. Scented oils set the mood by stimulated our all important olfactory nerves. The sense of smell is closely linked to areas of the brain that regulate the release of hormones, including sex hormones.

When choosing essential oils use pure oils from a health food store or order them from a high quality aromatherapy manufacturer. Commercial products that contain chemicals and fillers are often labeled as aromatherapy, but they are not the best choice. Read the label carefully and look out for other ingredients such as propylene glycol, artificial colors, and other chemical additives.

Essential Oil Use

All of these oils are known for their aphrodisiac properties: Ylang-ylang, sandalwood, patchouli, rose, musk, jasmine and vanilla.

- Rub a few drops of oil on a light bulb before turning on the light; or
- Fill a 2-ounce spritzer bottle with spring water, add 5 drops of each oil or any combination of the ones you enjoy. Spray around the room, and on yourself; or
- Add 5 to 10 drops of any combination of these oils to a warm bath; or
- For direct massage, add a few drops of essential oil to a base oil such as sesame or almond oil. (The essential oils are too strong to put directly on the skin, especially delicate mucus membranes.)

Lubricants

The best sexual lubricant is natural vaginal secretions. Saliva also works well. When more lubrication is needed, there are many water-based commercial lubricants on the market. However, many of them tend to dry up very quickly. Here are two oil based products that I have found to work quite well as sexual lubricants:

- *Aura Glow Almond Scent* by Heritage Products. This is an all-natural massage oil that works very well as an overall skin moisturizer. It is safe to use intra-vaginally. It is available in health food stores.
- *Albolene Liquifying Cleanser* works well as a sexual lubricant for occasional use. It contains mineral oil and paraffin, so it is not all natural, but it is long lasting and effective.

CHAPTER SEVEN

Menopause
Menopausal Moods

Menopause is defined as the cessation of the menstrual cycle, and is confirmed if no menstruation occurs for one year. Many cultures consider this an honor and a sign of great wisdom. The concept of the Crone as healer surfaces in many folkloric tales. Yet, in our youth glorifying culture menopause has taken on the status of a sign of aging with negative consequences—the loss of vitality, attractiveness, and sexuality. However, as we move forward in the new millennium, many vital, dynamic women entering their menopausal years are choosing to welcome this cycle of life with open arms and a positive attitude. They are viewing it as truly the golden years of mature adulthood. The North American Menopause Society (see www.menopause.org) conducted a poll that points to a changing attitude towards this change of life. Sixty percent of the women questioned thought they were just as attractive and dynamic after menopause, as they were before and 80 percent felt relieved that they no longer got their period.

CYCLES OF LIFE

The ending of the menstrual cycle is actually a culmination of a five- to ten-year period that precedes this event which can be filled with annoying and seemingly endless health issues; all part of a subdivision of time in the female life cycle called perimenopause.

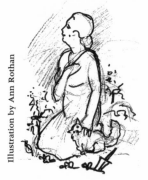

Illustration by Ann Rothan

Although the following discussion of symptoms may appear daunting, keep in mind that many woman do not experience any of them, and there is a great deal of individual differences as to the intensity of symptoms. Don't forget that there are also many positive health benefits that can come with menopause. If a woman has uterine fibroids, cystic breasts or endometriosis, these conditions often resolve themselves along with cessation of the menses.

THE SYMPTOMS OF MENOPAUSE

The experiences that women have during menopause seem to have a genetic tendency. Women will often experience symptoms at a similar age and with a similar degree of intensity as their mothers and grandmothers. As mentioned before, intensity can vary widely. For instance, although 75 percent of American women claim to have felt a hot flash (that number is as low as 25 percent in Japan), the number of hot flashes women experience can vary from one to hundreds of times, may last from a month to ten years, and be mildly annoying to quite devastating.

Many woman complain of having difficulty with recall, especially of recent events and small details. This is especially worrisome to the professional who relies on these abilities for her livelihood. This problem has earned the affectionate term of "having a senior moment." Insomnia, sleep difficulties, and mood swings are also quite common. Sexual appetite is often diminished, with a further complication of vaginal dryness and overall thinning of the vaginal walls leading to discomfort or pain during intercourse. Hot flashes are one the more dramatic signs, where a woman experiences a feeling of sudden heat throughout her body. She will often break into a mild to severe sweat which can be quite uncomfortable and embarrassing, especially when this happens in public. Hot flashes often occur while sleeping, followed by night sweats. It is interesting to note that many indigenous cultures have no reports of such occurrences, and in fact have no word in their language for hot flash. The leaching of bone, leading to the serious condition of osteoporosis, may develop after menopause and has been linked to decreased levels of estrogen and progesterone. Other symptoms may include mild to moderate depression, weight gain, changes in the regularity and amount of menstrual flow, and muscle and joint pain.

TREATING THE SYMPTOMS OF MENOPAUSE

Conventional Hormone Replacement Therapy (HRT)

Conventional medicine routinely prescribes hormone replacement therapy (HRT)—estrogen, often along with progestin, a synthetic form of progesterone, to help with many of the symptoms mentioned above. However, due to possible side effects, especially the threat of cancer, many women choose not to use it. A study presented in the *Journal of the American Medical Association* (January, 2000) reported a 40 percent increase in breast cancer among women taking estrogen (estradiol) along with progestin. Also, if you have a preexisting history of heart disease, cancer, circulatory problems, or high blood pressure, you may not be considered a candidate for HRT.

Designer Hormone Therapy

In holistic medicine we take a more prudent path—recommending a complete lifestyle program involving nutritious foods, exercise, stress reduction techniques, and the use of specific nutritional supplements and herbs. In a vast majority of woman these practices will effectively control and help to deal with all phases of transition experienced during menopause. In the few cases where it does not help to an acceptable degree, we will formulate a designer hormone formula. These are available via prescription through a compounding pharmacy, where the individualized prescription is prepared for the patient. First the holistic physician will order a battery of hormone tests to determine baseline levels of several hormones including: estradiol, estrone, estriol, progesterone, testosterone, and DHEA (dehydroepiandrosterone). A special formulation is then prepared which meets the individual woman's needs. In the HRT prescribed by conventional medicine the only form of estrogen used is estradiol . This kind of estrogen helps with memory and decreases hot flashes; however, estradiol is an aggressive form of estrogen linked to the increase in certain forms of cancer. It is often combined with progestin, an artificial form of progesterone, also linked to many unwanted side effects. The addition of progestin may decrease the risk of endometrial cancer, but increases the risk of breast cancer. The compounded formula prescribed by holistic physicians is quite different. It is a combination of all of the hormones in their natural form, which are often extracted from plant sources. It can be in either oral tablet form or mixed into a non-toxic cream base which is then applied directly to the skin and sometimes the vaginal tissues. This is called transdermal application—a delivery system that is particularly effective because hormones are *lipophilic,* "fat-loving" substances. They are easily absorbed by the fatty layers of the skin and are directly taken into the circulatory system.

Diet and Exercise

Many women report a marked decrease in hot flashes, mood swings, mental spaciness, and sexual doldrums by moving to an organic, vegetable-based diet, and including daily exercise in their life routines. Women who have been eating this way and exercising for years have reported decreased symptoms of menopause. Organic foods are vitally important because eating them is the only way to insure a limited intake of xenoestrogenic compounds, which play havoc with an already challenged hormonal balance. Xenoestrogens proliferate via pesticides and herbicides which are found in all non-organic food sources. Inorganic foods are also contaminated with genetically modified material. Since no research has been done on the long-term effect of genetically modified foods, it is prudent to avoid eating them. Decrease consumption of sugars, all artificial sweeteners (stevia is a great herbal sweetener), breads, and other wheat products, dairy products, and all fried foods. Increase consumption of dark green leafy vegetables, especially kale. These dietary suggestions will not only aid menopausal symptoms, but will decrease the likelihood of developing other degenerative illnesses associated with aging.[12]

Phytoestrogens

Foods that are high in phytoestrogens are particularly helpful. Phytoestrogens are plant derived substances that are molecularly similar to human estrogen. These are protective substances that can fit into the estrogen receptor sites in the body and block the uptake of more aggressive carcinogenic estrogens such as xenoestrogens and estradiol. Soy can make such a profound change that many women notice a decrease in perimenopausal symptoms by simply adding 1 ounce of Tofu and one 8-ounce glass of soymilk to their daily diet. Increasing essential fatty acids, especially omega-3 oils, is also important. Freshly ground flaxseed (1 to 2 tablespoons) sprinkled on food or flaxseed oil (2 tablespoons) can help to increase omega-3 levels. EPA-DHA from cold water fish such as salmon or mackerel is another source of these oils. Purslane is a common garden weed that is very high in omega-3 fatty acids.[13] Learn to identify it and use it in salads and soups.

Herbs

Along with cleaning up the diet and a commitment to daily exercise, herbs are wonderful natural adjunctive therapies to aid the body throughout menopause.

- **Black cohosh** can help to relieve hot flashes and also act as a mild relaxant and sleep aid.
- **Siberian ginseng** lifts mild to moderate depression, especially when combined with **rose buds**. It also is an overall tonic and enhances energy.
- **Licorice root** has actual estrogenic effects and

supports the adrenal glands, which has a regulatory effect on all other hormones. It is also an anti-inflammatory for muscle/joint aches.

- **Dong quai** is a strong phytoestrogen. It can help normalize menstrual irregularities, but may cause an increase in bleeding, so don't use it if heavy periods are a problem.
- **Chaste tree berry** *(Agnus castus, Vitex)* is one of the most helpful herbs for easing symptoms including hot flashes, fluid retention, and mild depression.
- **Wild yam** helps to increase the body's natural production of progesterone. It is often available as a cream, and is most effective if combined along with other ingredients such as pregnenelone and DHEA.
- **Nettles** are extremely nutritious and furnish much needed nutrients and minerals.
- **Sea vegetables** are high in minerals that support hormone formation. Sea vegetables are appropriate for all phases of the female cycle.
- **Motherwort** helps with hot flashes, irritability, heart palpitations, and other menopausal symptoms.

Chinese Medicine Approach to Menopause

The ancient practice of Chinese Medicine has relied on herbs for centuries to help women go through the change of life smoothly. Chinese practitioners provide a balanced approach of nutrition and herbs along with energy balancing techniques of acupuncture and acupressure.

The following is reprinted with permission from *New Living* magazine (1999):

Menopause

TRADITIONAL CHINESE MEDICINE
by Dr. Shauyon Liu

The premise of traditional Chinese medicine (TCM) is based on a holistic approach that seeks to balance the yin-yang energy of the body using acupuncture, acupressure, and herbs. Acupuncture is based on balancing the flow of chi, or life force energy of the body, by inserting fine needles into specific points that correlate to specific health problems in the body. These points have been mapped by the Chinese over a period of two thousand years and recent research using electromagnetics have confirmed their locations.

Stagnant energy, or blockages along these points caused by poor nutrition, stress, injury, illness, or not exercising enough, cause dysfunction in the body's organs eventually resulting in disease and pain. Only disposable acupuncture needles are used and because they are so fine, they are barely noticed by the patient upon their insertion. Acupressure is similar to massage except certain pressure points along the meridians of the body are stimulated by applying pressure and massage to reactivate the flow of chi.

The use of Chinese herbs combined with acupuncture and acupressure balance the chi in the body, easing depression, insomnia, irritability, anxiety, hot flashes, and other symptoms associated with menopause. Herbs that are tonics strengthen various organs and generally balance the flow of energy in the body. The kidney is important in Chinese medicine because the body's main source of energy emanates from this organ. Other herbs balance the yin (passive energy) or yang (active energy) of organs in the body. Herbs are also used as food in TCM in providing important nutrients. Chinese herbs that are helpful in alleviating the symptoms of menopause include:

Suan Zao Ren (wild Chinese jujube): a tonic, nutritive, and sedative that is important in drawing out the powers and energies of other herbs; it tonifies the spleen, retards aging, and is nourishing to the blood. Jujubes are said to clear the nine openings or apertures that connect human beings to the external world (these nine apertures are the: mouth, eyes, ears, nostrils, genitals, and anus). Jujubes help facilitate the smooth flow of energy through these apertures and along the meridians of the body.

71

Yuan Zhi (Polygala tenuifolia): a tonic, analgesic, and sedative that is important for the kidney, heart, and lungs; it increases muscle mass and prevents bone loss (important for preventing osteoporosis) and is a great overall mental health herb similar to St. John's wort; it promotes mental clarity while alleviating insomnia, depression, and anxiety.

Tain Ma (Gastrodia elata): The rhizome of this plant is used to balance the liver since a menopausal woman's fluctuating hormones tax the energy of the liver and throw it into overdrive as it works extra hard to detoxify all the hormones in the blood. It is also good at alleviating headaches and other mood imbalances.

San Qi (Pseudoginseng radix) is another liver-balancing herb that specifically works as a hemostatic herb to stop heavy bleeding and promote rapid healing; it tastes similar to ginseng (hence the pharmaceutical name) and was given the knickname "gold-no-trade" by the Chinese militia and martial artists who would not trade this lifesaving herb for all of the gold in China.

He Huan Pi (Albizziae cortex) is a heart and liver tonic primarily used to treat depression, insomnia, and irritability. Made from the bark of the Mimosa tree, this herb also strengthens the blood and reduces swelling. Sometimes He Huan Pi is combined with Chinese angelica root **(Dong quai)**, the "great tonic for all female deficiencies," to relieve pain; angelica is a great yin tonic while ginseng is a great yang tonic; sometimes He Haun Pi is combined with dandelion and wild chrysanthemum flower to purify the blood.

Bo Dze Ren (Thuja orientalis): This useful tree is used to promote hair growth, is a decorative item in Oriental gardens, and is used to make traditional Chinese furniture. The kernels of its fruit serve as a nutritive, sedative and tonic for the heart, spleen, and liver. It is used to stop uterine bleeding and is sometimes combined with Mugwort, a very prolific weed.

Traditional Chinese medicine incorporates a holistic mind/body approach to wellness. Healing herbs, acupuncture, and acupressure all work together to balance the body's chi. Good nutrition, exercise, and healthy spiritual practice also have a key role to play in helping a woman through her change of life.

Part II

herbs

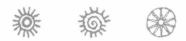

how to Prepare and Use herbs

HERBAL DELIVERY SYSTEMS

There are many delivery systems for herbs. In this section we will discuss several ways that herbs are commonly used: spices, teas, tinctures, extracts, capsules, oils, salves, suppositories, pessaries, poultices, compresses, and essential oils. All of these delivery systems can vary greatly in the quality of the product that they provide, depending on the growing conditions of the plants, care in processing, and scientific quality control of the finished product. We'll include a discussion about the current trend of standardization by the herbal industry.

Spices

Spices are herbs added to food. In most cultures it is a culinary practice to add flavor and color to foods. But spices often have health benefits, such as bitters aiding digestion or hot spices discouraging parasites. When using herbs as spices, either grow your own or buy organic varieties. Commercially available non-organic spices are irradiated, decreasing both their nutritional and medicinal value; it also severely cuts down on their flavor. (Test this for yourself by comparing the taste of a commercial and organic brand of any common spice such as thyme, rosemary, or garlic powder!)

Teas

Infusions

An infusion is a tea made from plant parts. Tea is an ancient method of preparing herbs as medicine and is as useful today as it was in times past. Teas are inexpensive and can be easily prepared at home from garden grown or wildcrafted herbs. Teas can also be made from bulk dried or fresh herbs purchased from a grocery or health food store. Health food stores now carry a variety of teas that combine several herbs into medicinal formulas. *Longlife* and *Traditional Medicinals* are two of the many excellent brands that are available. To make an infusion use 1 teaspoon ground or chopped leaf, flower, or herbaceous stem for each 1 cup of water. Pour boiling water on plant parts. Allow to steep for 5 to 10 minutes. If bitter herbs are used, more flavorful herbs such as licorice, peppermint, or the herbal sweetener stevia can be added to mask the bitter flavor. An infusion will extract many water soluble active constituents from plants, but is the weakest form of medicinally prepared herbs. It is also less likely to cause any kind of adverse reactions when compared to more concentrated preparations. The potency of infusions varies tremendously due to differences in preparation and strength of the herbs used, which diminishes the possibility of knowing the exact dose of medicinal constituents derived from teas. Using teas to treat a particular condition may be inconvenient because a lot of tea may need to be ingested (4 to 10 cups a day). Besides, modern women may not have time to make tea on the go. Also, a standardized dose cannot be guaranteed.

Aside from the inconveniences, this method of administering herbs has been used throughout history with excellent results! Herbal teas can be used as a healthy daily habit, while more concentrated herbs can be used for specific conditions.

SUN TEA

Sun tea delights both children and adults! Pour filtered water into a large glass jar. Add either fresh or dried plant parts or prepared herbal tea bags, about 1 teaspoon herbs to 1 cup of water. Place jar outside or on a window sill in a sunny location and allow to steep for several hours. Drink at room temperature or refrigerate and drink cold with ice.

Decoctions

Decoctions are also herb teas but are more concentrated and prepared differently. Parts of plants that tend to be more solid such as roots, bark, stems, and seeds need to be cut up into small pieces and simmered in order to extract the active ingredients. Simmering continues from 20 minutes to up to several hours with some types of plants. The water is allowed to evaporate to increase the concentration of the decoction. Decoctions can be preserved for later use by storing in the refrigerator or adding 20 percent alcohol.

Tinctures and Extracts

These are liquid preparations. Liquids have the advantage of being easier to swallow, which is especially helpful for young children, the elderly, and those who find swallowing pills difficult. Also, several liquids can easily be taken at once, by putting them all into juice or tea. The active herbal constituents in liquids may be absorbed more easily by the body since they are already in liquid form and don't require additional digestion. Both of these preparations are made by soaking plant parts in a *menstruum*—a solvent used to extract active constituents. Alcohol is the most common menstruum. Other substances used for extraction include apple cider vinegar and glycerin. Modern pharmaceutical practices include the use of benzene and other toxic chemicals, along with high heat, to extract medicinal components. We do not recommend products that are manufactured in this manner. The herb manufacturers mentioned in the back of this book use only natural methods for extraction. The percentage of alcohol needed varies according to the plant and the desired components. For instance, the oil resins in peppermint require more alcohol than water soluble substances. The strength of a tincture is usually 1:5, which means there is one part active herbal component to 5 parts of solution. Extracts are processed further to concentrate the active component to a 1:1 ratio. Although alcohol is an excellent preservative, alcohol-free extracts may be preferable because some individuals dislike the strong taste of alcohol. Alcohol can also stress a weakened or underfunctioning liver in sensitive people and those suffering from allergies, environmental sensitivities, systemic candida (yeast infections), and a host of other health concerns. Of course, people in recovery from alcoholism should avoid extracts with alcohol, as should young children. Read labels carefully. An extract with 1:1 ratios and no toxic additives is the best choice.

MAKE YOUR OWN TINCTURE

Place freshly collected leaves, flowers, and/or herbaceous stems into a large glass jar. Cover completely with alcohol. Some states sell 200 proof (100 percent) alcohol. If that is not available vodka works well. Allow herbs to continue to soak for 1 to 2 months. Shake mixture every day or so. Strain finished tincture into an amber glass jar. It will remain potent for several years if kept in a cool, dry place. Remember to label the finished product.

Capsules

Capsules are made by drying and pulverizing herbal materials into a powder. The powder is then placed in gelatin capsules, which makes it easier to swallow. Capsules may be made from a single herb or a combination of herbs. As with all herbal preparations, these vary as to quality depending on the process and raw materials used by the manufacturer. Some capsules are standardized and others are not. Read labels, including the inactive ingredients, to be aware of what the capsule contains. Capsules may be more convenient for the herbal user on the go since a daily dose can be packed in a pill carrier. Capsules also override the sometimes bitter and unpleasant flavors associated with some kinds of herbs, and are the least messy to take.

MAKE YOUR OWN CAPSULES

Use your own wild-crafted or cultivated herbs or buy bulk herbs purchased from a health food store (*Frontier* offers a large variety). Dry the herbs thoroughly. Hang fresh herbs upside down by tying the ends together with dental floss or string and hanging them out of the sun in a totally dry basement or closet. Another good drying method is to spread the herbs out in a single layer on paper towels in a dry, low-light area. When dry, grind them into a powder using a mortar and pestle or electric coffee grinder. Empty gelatin capsules are available at most health food stores. Vegetarian capsules called "vegicaps" are also available. Pack the capsules with the dried powder. Manual capsule packers can be purchased if you feel you will be making a lot of capsules. Of course, you can always choose commercially prepared capsules. (After preparing your own capsules, you will appreciate the cost effectiveness of commercially prepared ones.)

Oils

Herbs can be soaked in oil in the sun to extract fat-soluble components. Herbal oils can be used topically for skin conditions. Comfrey, chickweed, and St. John's wort are a few of the plants that can be used to make herbal oils.

ST. JOHN'S WORT OIL

Gather St. John's wort when it is in full flower, near June 24—St. John's Day in England. Check the yellow flower tops for tiny black dots; it may be helpful to use a magnifying glass. The black dots contain hypericin—one of the active ingredients. Use good quality oil as a base, sesame or olive oil work well. Fill a glass jar with flowers and leaves. Cover with oil. Leave the jar on a windowsill or on the dashboard of your car. After a few days you will notice that the yellow flowers are fading, but the oil is turning a bright red. Allow the mixture to sit for at least one week, then strain out the flower parts. Add 1 teaspoon of vitamin E for each pint of oil to act as a preservative. You may want to keep the oil in the refrigerator to increase its shelf life. St. John's wort oil has a soothing, anti-pain effect. It can be used on sore muscles or over the uterus for menstrual or postpartum pains. It also has anti-viral properties and can be soothing to skin abrasions and injuries. Use it as a scalp rub along with a few drops of tea tree oil to relieve dandruff.

Salves

Salves are like oils except that beeswax is added to make a semi-solid substance that sticks to the skin like petroleum jelly. Salves are soothing and stay in place longer than oils. The beeswax adds to the overall healing effects.

HEALING SKIN SALVE

The following herbs can be grown in your garden, found in the wild, or purchased at a health food store.

> Use all or some of these herbs:
>> Lavender
>> Pine needles
>> Comfrey (leaves and roots)
>> Jewelweed
>> Aloe vera leaf
>> Rose petals
>> Rosemary
> Olive or coconut oil
> Pure beeswax (2 ounces of wax per 1 cup of oil)
> Vitamin E (½ tsp per 1 cup of oil)

Chop all ingredients and then mix together with a mortar and pestle. Place mixture in a deep pan; use enough oil to completely cover the herbal mixture. *Slowly* heat the oil over low heat, stirring for one hour. Do not fry or allow to smoke. Press the herbal mixture often to squeeze out active ingredients. Strain into a glass or stainless steel pot or container. Melt the beeswax; add melted wax to the strained oil and mix thoroughly. Add vitamin E as a preservative. Pour into small jars and allow to cool and solidify. Keep refrigerated.

This recipe will produce the best skin salve available. I have seen it instantly heal small wounds—to the amazement of the injured party. It will smooth skin and decrease wrinkles. Add a few drops of essential oils to the mixture for variation and aroma enhancement.

Suppositories and Pessaries

These are delivered into the body through the rectum or vagina. Suppositories and pessaries increase absorption of medicinal components since they are not broken down by digestive juices. Americans rarely use suppositories, but they are common in Europe and other parts of the world. My friend is a physician in St. Martin. He often cares for American tourists. One woman came to him complaining of an ear infection. He prepared an anti-microbial herbal suppository and told her to return in two days. When he examined her ear again, it was oozing with an oily liquid. He had taken for granted that everyone knows where a suppository goes, and had not given her specific instructions on how to use it—she had stuck it in her ear!

MAKING AN HERBAL PESSARY:

Cocoa Butter (available in health food stores)
Desired herbs

Herbs can be used as dry powder (1 teaspoon), extract (30 drops), or essential oil (2 drops) for each tablespoon of cocoa butter. Various combinations of herbs can be used depending on the therapeutic effect desired.

YEAST INFECTION PESSARY:

Goldenseal or Oregon graperoot
¼ tsp garlic powder
Powdered acidophilus
Tea tree oil

Blend all ingredients into cocoa butter. Place this mixture on a sheet of wax paper. Roll into small logs about half the size of a tampon. Place in freezer to harden. Once hard, store up to one week in refrigerator. Insert one per day in the evening.

Poultices

Poultices are preparations made from herbs and then applied to the skin. Poultices, such as a mustard pack, were a very common form of home remedy in most cultures, including the United States, up until the last half of the twentieth century. Herbal poultices use a base to create a thick substance that can easily stick to the skin. Common bases include ground flaxseeds, grated potatoes or onions, slippery elm powder, agar-agar, oatmeal, cornmeal, or flour.

FACIAL POULTICE

½ cup oatmeal
1 fresh comfrey leaf, 1 Tbs dried powdered leaf, or 20 drops tincture
½ teaspoon dried green tea powder
1 egg white

Mix all ingredients together. Add enough warm water (or milk) to create a paste. Spread on face,cover with warm wet washcloth, and leave on for 15 minutes. Rinse.

Compresses

Compresses are made by soaking a cloth in a strong herbal tea and then applying it directly to the skin. It is often used for painful areas or skin problems.

HERBS IN A STOCKING COMPRESS

Gather fresh aromatic herbs or use dried bulk herbs. Peppermint, scented geranium, lavender, and rose all work well; or use any other scented herb or flower you enjoy. Place all herbs in a cut off or knee-high stocking. Put stocking around bathtub faucet and fasten with a rubber band. Allow hot water to run through until bath is almost full. Add enough cold water to bring water to a comfortable temperature. Soak for 20 minutes and use the stocking as an herbal body scrub.

Essential Oils

Essential oils are very different from herbal oils. While herbal oils are made by simply soaking an herb in oil, essential oils are derived through distillation. It is a long arduous process that yields a small amount of oil from a large batch of raw materials, thus the pricey cost of good quality essential oils. The therapeutic use of essential oils is called aromatherapy. It is an entire subdivision within the larger theater of herbal medicine that focuses on the medicinal use of essential oils to treat the mental, emotional, and physical aspects of the self. Essential oils should be mixed with a mild base oil, such as almond oil, when applied directly to the skin. Essential oils are often used as inhalants. Commercial diffusers are available or simply sprinkle a few drops of oil on a light bulb or at the bottom of your shower. Essential oils have myriad effects on the totality of the human being. The effects include stimulation of the olfactory nerve, which leads to emotion centers in the brain. This is why certain aromas stimulate particular feelings. However, the therapeutic value of aromatherapy goes way beyond the sense of smell, alone. Active chemical compounds in many oils can have specific effects, such as muscular relaxation, reduction of inflammation, and antibacterial properties. The benefits of the oils can be quite profound since the herbal components are delivered directly into the circulatory system through the skin. This reduces the breakdown of active ingredients that occurs during digestion. Oils are lipophilic or fat-loving, which makes it easy for them to be absorbed by the skin.

MENSTRUAL OR POSTPARTUM PAIN ESSENTIAL OIL RUB

1 oz. almond or sesame oil
2 drops clary sage oil
2 drops angelica oil
2 drops St. John's wort oil
2 drops lavender oil

Pour the almond or sesame oil into a small cup. Sprinkle in two drops each of any or all of the herb oils. (Be sure to purchase them from a high quality manufacturer—see Resources, page 185.) Rub on area over the uterus and on the lower back for a relaxing effect. You can add wild yam cream and castor oil to this combination. Cover area with a washcloth soaked in warm water or a hot water bottle for additional pain relief.

Botanical Medical Preparations Quick Reference Guide

From *The Natural Medicine Chest* by Eugene R. Zampieron
and Ellen Kamhi (New York: M. Evans, 1999).

Form		Strength
Infusion	A tea made by pouring hot water over flowers or leaves and allowing mixture to steep, covered, for 5 to 30 minutes	1:20
Decoction	A tea made from barks, roots, seeds, and stems, in which the water is gently simmered, covered, for 10 minutes to several hours.	1:10
Tincture	Alcohol (or another solvent) is poured over macerated (cut up and pulverized) plant parts. This mixture is then tightly covered, periodically shaken, and allowed to sit in a dark, cool area for several weeks to several months.	1:5
Extract (fluid)	The alcohol solvent is removed from the tincture, increasing the concentration.	1:1
Extract (solid)	The fluid extract is further concentrated, creating a tar or paste.	4:1 to 100:1
Tablets	This form may contain powdered herbs or solid extract materials. The strength can vary greatly, so be sure to check the labels.	Varies
Poultice	An external application of one herb or a combination of herbs mashed together. A poultice is often accompanied by heat, such as a heating pad or hot water bottle.	Varies
Herbal oil	Herbs soaked in oil produce an oil containing the medicinal components of the herbs. This form is used as a topical application	Varies
Herbal salve	Herbs are heated in oil and then pressed out. The oil is mixed with beeswax to produce a topical form.	Varies

CONGESTION RELIEF ESSENTIAL OIL INHALANT

5 to 10 drops eucalyptus oil
5 to 10 drops lemon oil

Close windows and vents in your bathroom and run the shower on maximum hot while you sit on toilet or bathtub. Once the room starts to steam, sprinkle ten drops of each oil on the bottom of the shower. Inhale steam.

Or, sprinkle five to ten drops of each oil in a small pot of boiling water. Remove the pot from the stove and place in a secure position on the counter. Cover head and pot with a towel. Breathe in steam. Be sure to stay far enough back to avoid steam burns.

After making your own herbal medicines, you will be a better judge of the commercial varieties since you will be intimately familiar with aroma, texture, color, and other attributes of herbal preparations.

STANDARDIZED VS. NON-STANDARDIZED HERBS

When we enter a health food store we are barraged by a multitude of herbal products. To add to the confusion some herbal products claim to be standardized while others do not. Standardization refers to the creation of an herbal product that contains a guaranteed potency of a particular compound found in an herb. Standardization surfaced in the European marketplace in 1992. It was developed by manufacturers interested in delivering guaranteed potency products to physicians who regularly use herbs in their practice, which is common in Europe and most of the world with the exception of the United States. These physicians and other researchers wanted to be certain of the exact dose of medicinal components that patients received each time they used an herb. Standardization begins with an analysis of the chemical compounds present in plant material. This is accomplished through the use of various techniques such as chromatography, spectrophotometry, and MRIs. Through years of scientific research a particular plant compound (or group of compounds) is often found to produce a specific desired medicinal effect. Each batch of product produced can then be tested to ensure that it contains a specific amount of that particular chemical compound. If it does not, additional portions of the active compound may be added.

Standardization has many benefits including:

- increased knowledge about the best way to grow and harvest herbs for maximum medicinal benefit
- consistency in manufacturing processes
- administration of more exact dosing

However, standardization can also have some downsides. For instance, ongoing research can discover additional compounds with active effects not previously understood. Different manufacturers may choose different chemical constituents to use as the basis of standardization. Also, just because a product is standardized does not mean it is pure and of the best quality. Some companies offer standardized herbal products that also contain artificial coatings, dyes, fillers, and binders. (Be sure to read the label information listed as "other ingredients.") Standardization may entirely miss the idea that for maximum health benefits extracts should retain as many of the natural constituents found in the plant, in the same ratios found in nature, as possible. In many instances, due to chemical complexity and lack of in depth research, it is not yet known how constituents within a plant work together to provide a specific physiological effect. Also, although a constituent may have been identified as being key to the herb's medicinal effect (*e.g.*, hypericin in St. John's wort), this may be misleading because we don't know how other components aid the known active ingredient to generate an overall positive effect. For instance, another compound, *hyperforin*, is now thought to be involved in St. John's wort's activity. One fact stands clear: herbs have been used by mankind as medicine for thousands of years without the benefit of standardization. Standardization can be used as a modern guideline while we continue to honor the whole plant concept.

HERB/PHARMACEUTICAL
DRUG INTERACTIONS

The interaction between herbs and prescription or over-the-counter drugs is a serious and growing concern. Drugs did not exist during most of the many thousands of years that herbs have been used as medicine, except in very recent history. During the later part of the 1900s (1960–1996) most of the people who used herbs did *not* use pharmaceutical drugs. However, following the national media coverage of St. John's wort in 1996, the use of herbs suddenly was catapulted into mainstream culture. Now, a vast number of people are retuning to the use of herbs. Mainstream physicians are also beginning to integrate herbs into their treatment protocols. As this trend continues, the possibility of negative effects due to drug/herb interactions becomes more of an issue.

It is outside the scope of this book to delve into specific herb-drug interactions. However, cautions are indicated following the discussion of each herb. A good source for checking the most current research on herb/drug interactions is the American Botanical Council (see www.herbalgram.org). If you are on prescription medications be sure to consult a knowledgeable health care practitioner before using herbs.

CHAPTER NINE

herbs

Our Plant Sisters

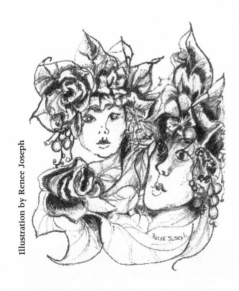

Illustration by Renee Joseph

The herbs discussed in this chapter are often used to help balance women's health issues. These herbs are referred to elsewhere in this book, but in this chapter we will explore each of the herbs more deeply. We will delve into their history and folklore and give you specific recommendations for dosing.

CYCLES OF LIFE

Black Cohosh (Cimicifuga racemosa)

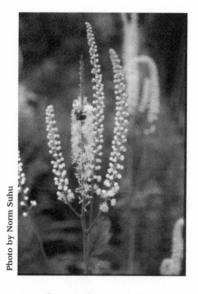

Photo by Norm Suhu

The black cohosh plant is a perennial bush in the buttercup family that can grow up to nine feet high. It is found in woodlands throughout the Northeast. The root is the part that is used medicinally. The best time to collect the roots is in the autumn after the fruits have ripened. The roots can be sliced along the long axis and dried with care to avoid the formation of mold.

The plant has several common names which reflect the many uses that have been attributed to it, including "snakeroot," "bugbane," "rattleweed" and "squawroot." *Cohosh* is a Native American Algonquin word that refers to the rough surface of the root structures, called rhizomes. "Snakeroot" reflects its use as a snakebite remedy. "Bugbane" comes from the ability of the plant's odor to repel insects. In Europe the flowers were stuffed into pillows for this purpose. When the dry seeds found on the plants in late fall are blown by the wind, they rattle, thus "rattleweed." Several native cultures used the rattling of the plant for their sacred ceremonies. Black cohosh was also called "squawroot" because it was commonly used by Native Americans to assist in all manner of women's ailments including scanty, heavy, painful, and irregular menstrual flow; inability to conceive; and menopausal symptoms such as hot flashes and vaginal dry-ness. The Iriquois reportedly used it to increase milk flow.

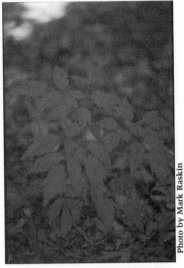

Black cohosh root extract was reg-ularly recommended by the Eclectic physicians in the mid 1800s for mus-cle aches and pains and other rheu-matic complaints, as a mild sedative for insomnia, and for all female com-plaints. *The Kings American Dispen-satory* refers to black cohosh as a "very active, powerful and useful remedy."

Black cohosh is among an ever growing group of herbs where mod-ern scientific analysis reveals the chemical constituents that help to explain the longtime observations of herbalists throughout his-tory. The extract contains glycosides and isoflavones which may impart an estrogenic effect. One specific isoflavone, formononetin, was shown to be able to bind to estrogen receptor sites *in vitro* (in a test tube). One study demonstrated that black cohosh measura-bly lowered luteinizing hormone (LH) levels in menopausal women.[14] Hot flashes are attributed in part to a decrease in estro-gen production and an increase in LH levels in menopausal women. At least one animal study suggests that black cohosh may be useful in preventing osteoporosis.

Black cohosh should *not* be used during pregnancy, but it can be very helpful if used right before delivery. As we see with many herbs, black cohosh can have a normalizing effect depending on what the body needs at the time. If false labor (Braxton-Hicks con-tractions) occurs, black cohosh relaxes the uterus and eases the pain. However, if true labor has started, black cohosh increases the strength of the contractions and eases birth! It is also excellent to help with postpartum pain. Its sedative properties can also soothe the agitation and anxiety following labor.

Dosages

Tea made from dried root	3–4 cups/day
	(1 cup water to ½ tsp dried root)
Capsule	40 mg/day
Extract	½–1 ml/day

Black Cohosh may be standardized to 1 mg deoxyactin : 20 mg extract, or 2.5% triterpene glycosides—follow label directions on the brand you select.

Cautions

- Discontinue use during pregnancy.
- Headaches, dizziness, nausea, and visual disturbances have been reported after taking large amounts (over 3 grams/day).
- May potentiate the effect of antihypertensive medications.

Blue Cohosh
(Caulophyllum thalictroides)

Blue cohosh is an important botanical for women to consider using during childbirth years. It was used by the Algonquins as a remedy to correct menstrual disorders of all kinds, to prepare the uterus for childbirth, to speed labor, and as an analgesic remedy to ease both false and real labor pain.

This Native American herb is a kin of barberry (*Berberis vulgaris*) and Oregon grape root (*Berberis aquafolium*). It is a member of the family *Berberidaceae* and also contains the same types of berberine alkaloids and caulosaponins, compounds that can mimic the effect of steroids and reproductive hormones.

The leaves when young are a bluish purple, and as they mature the color turns into a rich blue-green hue, thus the name blue cohosh. The leaves resemble a three part hoofed foot, and the perennial plant thrives in the rich humus along streams which abound in the shade of North American eastern forests. Today it is not as plentiful due to years of over-harvesting. The root is dug in the autumn, dried, and made into a tea by simmering for an hour.

When the herb was rediscovered by the Eclectic physicians in the late 1800s, they wrote extensively on its ability to expedite childbirth, especially when labor had stopped or slowed due to weakness, fatigue associated with long labor, or uterine muscular weakness. It was used in place of oxytocin (a drug which causes strong uterine contractions) because of its gentle but effective nature. It was also given as a first resort when a forceps delivery was imminent, but could cause damage to the fetus.

John Uri Lloyd, one of the most brilliant pharmacologists of the

Eclectic era, did extensive studies on the herb and discovered that it contained high levels of potassium, magnesium, calcium, iron, silicon, and phosphorus, many of which are vital nutrients during pregnancy, especially to accommodate the rapid growth of the fetus during the last trimester. He also isolated one particular chemical compound, leontin, which he patented as a botanical drug to be used specifically in cases of ammenorrhea (lack of a menstrual period).

Blue cohosh is used as a strong tea {decoction} starting four to six weeks prior to the expected due date, or in the combination known as the "mother's cordial" or "MCHV" formula. This formula, which is still used by naturopathic physicians, midwives, and herbalists today, is composed of *Mitchella repens* (partridge berries), *Caulophyllum thalictriodes* (blue cohosh), *Helonis dioica* (false unicorn root), and *Viburnum opulus* (cramp bark). This formula strengthens and prepares the uterus for childbirth, and assists labor.

Dosage

Tincture	10–30 drops, 3×/day between meals

Cautions

Do not use in early pregnancy. Use at the end of the third trimester or the beginning of the ninth month of pregnancy, *only* with the supervision of a knowledgeable health care practitioner.

Burdock (Arctium lappa)

Burdock is found throughout the temperate zones around the world, often in vacant lots or along paths. It is a powerful plant that grows over two seasons. The first year the leaves stay close to the ground. This is the best time to gather the burdock root, which is used as a food staple in many areas of the world. (Whenever you are looking for the root of any plant, the best time to get it is when a lot of the plant's energy is concentrated in that area.) Early spring provides the best roots, especially for use by adolescents. However, to get the early spring roots you need to know where burdock grew the fall before. Mark the area with a stake or special rock and return to the same spot in the early spring. The fall is also a good time for root gathering because the plant stores nutrients in the root as it prepares to over winter. During the second season, the plant puts out a stalk that can grow quite tall, up to five feet. The stalk produces seeds, and the part of the plant that many people are familiar with—the burrs. These give burdock its name. If you have ever walked through the woods in the fall you may have found these stickies on your pants and socks or even matted into your dog's fur. Amazingly enough, one entrepreneurial gentleman developed the idea for Velcro from observing these burrs!

Burdock is a slow acting nutritional tonic that builds strength over time. It is highly nutritious and contains minerals such as magnesium, calcium, potassium, and silica. Burdock is considered an alterative or blood cleanser in herbal medicine. It aids the organs of detoxification and elimination such as the lymphatic system, skin, liver, kidneys, and digestive system. The uterus, which empties its contents each month (except during pregnancy), is an organ of elimination influenced by the action of burdock In Chinese medicine it is considered a cooling herb, useful for hot conditions such as hot flashes or swollen joints. It can help with frequent urinary tract infections and has diuretic properties. Cherokee women relied on burdock to strengthen the uterus and aid the birth process.

Obtain burdock by gathering the root yourself or purchasing the root in the oriental food sections of most grocery stores where it is called "gobo." It can be sliced and steamed or mixed along with veggies in a stir-fry. Burdock is an excellent addition to fresh vegetable juice. It is also available as a liquid extract or capsules in health food stores.

BURDOCK ACNE COMPRESS

Fresh burdock root
Oatmeal
Aloe vera juice

Grate the burdock and mix with oatmeal and enough aloe vera juice to make a paste. Put directly on affected area and leave on for about half an hour. Remove with lukewarm water.

You can use burdock internally as well, especially in combination with yellow dock and red clover as an alterative or blood cleanser.

Dosages

Fresh root	6 inches of root/day steeped as tea or juice
Extract	20 drops 3×/day
Capsules	2 caps (450–500 mg) 2×/day

Burning Bush (Dictamnus albus)

"Burning bush" and "white dittany" are two names for this plant that grows in mountainous regions of Europe, Asia and northern areas of the United States. It has heart-shaped leaves and a dramatic five-pointed-star seed pod which contains black seeds. Lemon scent glands cover the entire plant. They exude a volatile oil that creates a pleasant aroma during the summer. The leaf and pinkish flowers are prepared into a homeopathic remedy (*Flor albus*) used for women's health problems such as irregular periods and urinary complaints. The root has been used as a diuretic and causes the uterus to contract, thus leading to its use as a contraceptive and to promote menstruation.

	Dosage
Tea	½ teaspoon herb/2 cups of water 2–3 cups tea throughout the day

Caution

- Do not use during pregnancy.
- Burning bush may cause a rash if it touches the skin.

Cascara Sagrada (Rhamnus purshiana)

Cascara is a mild laxative with a long history of use. The name *cascara sagrada* means "sacred bark" in Spanish. It grows in the Pacific Northwest and was used by the indigenous First Nations People of that area for many centuries. By the 1890s it was a popular drug marketed by Parke-Davis and remains in use today, both as an herb and an over-the-counter pharmaceutical drug. To use cascara as a laxative the bark is stripped off the *Rhamnus purshiana* tree and must be allowed to dry for over one year before it is made into a medicament. It contains active compounds that increase peristalsis (the snake-like movement of the colon). It can also act as a stool softener by decreasing the amount of water absorbed via the large intestines.

Dosages

Liquid extract	10 drops once/day
Capsules	1–2 caps (400–500 mg) once/day as needed

Read all label directions carefully!

Caution

Laxatives must be used sparingly to avoid dependency. They may also cause potassium depletion if used in excess. Use only as often as necessary to offset constipation, never for more than seven to ten days at a time. Often one to three times per week is sufficient. Do not use while pregnant without a physician's supervision.

Castor Bean Plant/Castor Oil
(Ricinus communis)

The castor bean plant is called *Palma Christi*, or palm of Christ, due to the hand-like shape of its leaves and the widespread use for its healing properties. It grows around the world in tropical and subtropical areas. The castor bean itself contains ricin, a highly toxic compound that can be fatal. However, the oil pressed from the seeds is safe to use since pressing the oil removes the ricin. A castor oil pack is an extremely useful treatment for nonmalignant ovarian and breast cysts as well as for helping to remove 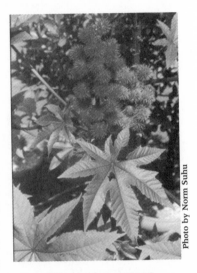 toxins through the skin. Dr. Forest Clinton Jarvis in his 1958 best-selling book *Folk Medicine* describes many uses of castor oil applied externally to the skin. "Apply it to moles, warts, and skin ulcers to remove or lesson the blemishes. Or rub a small amount on the hair and eye lashes to make them more luxuriant." Castor oil has been used historically as a laxative when taken orally. In general, its function is to drain toxins out of the body. I have personally seen small tumors, cysts, and other growths literally come out through the skin after a few days of application of castor oil. It is this same action which can cause a miscarriage if used in early pregnancy. Castor oil has been used historically to help induce labor at the termination of pregnancy. Current research substantiates this ancient claim.[15]

Dosages

Externally	apply as needed
Internally	½ to 1 tsp/day (occasional use only)

Cautions

- Do not use internally in early pregnancy.
- Discontinue internal use if it has a strong laxative effect.
- Do not use with obstruction, inflammatory intestinal disorders, or with abdominal pain.

CASTOR OIL PACK

Castor oil
Undyed flannel
Heating pad or hot water bottle
Plastic sheet or large plastic bag
Terrycloth towel
Ace bandage

Soak flannel with castor oil. Place flannel on area of body you wish to treat—do not use over uterus in early pregnancy. Cover flannel with plastic. Place heating pad or hot water bottle on pack-use heating pad on low setting—if the oil gets too hot, it may burn the skin. Secure in place with ace bandage. Leave the pack on the effected area for one half to two hours. Use it when you are going to sleep and then take it off during the night.

This treatment was recommended by Edgar Cayce, the famous psychic who lived in the 1940s. He suggested that it be used for ovarian cysts, fibroids, breast swellings, headaches, menstrual cramps, constipation, liver problems, and to hasten the elimination of toxins. It is soothing, relaxing, and increases circulation of blood, lymph, and chi (life force energy). Keep it handy and try it often!

Chamomile (Matricaria chamomilla, Anthemis noblis)

The latin name of this plant, *Matricaria,* means "mother of the gut." The stomach is often associated with emotional upset. For instance, the common expression, "I can't stomach that" usually means that something is upsetting to that person. Upset stomach, irritability, and insomnia are symptoms often experienced by girls in menarche, during PMS, and during menopause. Chamomile flowers are dainty and beautiful, emerging in early summer. The Doctrine of Signatures also reminds us of the springtime cycle of menarche. Chamomile flowers can be gathered from the garden and used 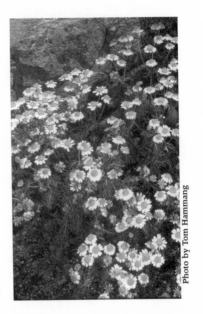 as a prepared tea, extract, or capsule. In fact chamomile tea is the most commonly used herbal beverage in the United States. Take a chamomile tea bag along in your purse or backpack, and just order hot water at your local diner. Used as a nightcap, it will help with digestion as well as a good night's sleep. Chamomile has active constituents that ease anxiety and muscle tension and have an overall calming effect.

Photo by Tom Hammang

Dosages	
Tea	1 tsp flowers to 1 cup water
	1–2 cups/day
Capsules	250 mg 2×/day

Cautions

- Chamomile can cause allergic reactions in those who are sensitive to ragweed pollen.
- Chamomile may have an additive effect with the drug wafarin.
- Do not use along with alcohol or benzodiazepines.

Chaste Tree Berry (Agnus castus, Vitex)

The chaste berry tree is indigenous to the Mediterranean area, although it can grow in temperate areas worldwide. It is an attractive bush with finger-like leaves and thin violet, blue, or pink flowers. The fruit produced by this tree is a dark brown-to-black berry, about the size of a peppercorn, with a spicy pepper flavor.

The chaste berry has a long history of use as an herbal medicine. It was first mentioned in the fourth century B.C. by Hippocrates, and was indicated in the King's American Dispensary as a remedy for female problems. It's common name reflects the belief that eating the fruit decreases sex drive and allows for increased chastity. During ancient Greek and Roman times, the priestess of the temple would eat the berries to lessen the libido. Another name for the plant, monk's pepper, came from the use by medieval monks towards a similar goal. Although scientific studies do not support the herb's ability to decrease sex drive, modern research shows that chaste berry has a regulating effect on the pituitary gland by

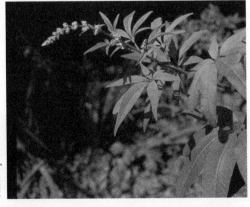

Photo by Norm Suhu

regulating the release of prolactin. Prolactin is a specific hormone which increases milk supply in a nursing mother, but also causes many menstrual irregularities in non-lactating women. Problems associated with high prolactin levels include PMS, infertility, scanty and heavy bleeding, endometriosis, and problems associated with menopause. Chaste berry has been the subject of in-depth placebo-controlled double blind studies, which have uncovered some of the specific mechanisms that make it so useful as a remedy for the female cycle. It has proven to be especially useful if irregularities are due to a deficiency in the formation of the corpus luteum in the ovaries. This yellow body is formed after ovulation and is responsible for the production of progesterone. Chaste berry increases the production of lutenizing hormone (LH) and decreases follicle-stimulating hormone (FSH). This enhances the ratio of progesterone to estrogen which helps regulate many hormone-based health problems. Chaste berries may need to be used for several months to elicit the desired effect. Please note that this herbal remedy is often called "agnus castus" or "vitex."

Dosages

Tea	1 tsp fresh or dried berries to 1 cup water, steeped for 10 minutes 1–2 cups/day
Extract	10–40 drops 2×/day
Capsules	1 cap (40 mg) 1×/day

Cautions

Do not use during pregnancy. If using chaste berry to enhance fertility, discontinue use once conception has occurred. Do not use along with birth control pills or other prescription hormone therapies. The use of chaste tree berry rarely has any negative effects, although in a small percentage of users skin rashes and increased menstrual flow have been reported.

Damiana
(Turnera aphrodisiaca, diffusa)

Damiana is a low growing shrub with yellow flowers and smooth green oval leaves. The leaves are the medicinal part of the plant. They are picked while the flowers are blooming. The fruit has a distinctive aroma, exudes a resinous substance, and contains yellow crescent-shaped seeds. The shrub is native to Central America and has a long history of use as an herbal medicine in Mexico, dating back to the ancient Aztec and Mayan civilizations. It is also found growing in Texas, the Caribbean, and southern Africa.

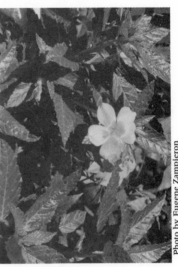

Photo by Eugene Zampieron

Chemical analysis has revealed various chemical constituents including volatile oils (terpenes), glycosides (such as arbutin—known to have antimicrobial activities), the bitter substance damianin, and beta-sitosterol, a phytosterol that may be involved with its effects on the sexual organs.

Damiana is a helpful tonic for the nervous system, the genito-urinary tract, and the kidneys, and is used for its abilities to tone the mucus membranes of the reproductive organs. Notice its species name—*aphrodisiaca*. This speaks of the most renowned use of this herb—as an aphrodisiac and sexual stimulant for both sexes. Damiana is an antidepressant and is used to increase libido.

In Jamaican folk medicine it is called *ram goat dash along*, because when male goats eat it, their libido increases dramatically!

Its ability to promote a euphoric state if taken in sufficient quantities was used by shamans during rituals because it helped to break inhibitions and promote the feeling of astral travel—to explore spiritual dimensions.

Damiana is the name of a commercial liquor produced in Mexico from this same plant. Some claim that the aphrodisiac properties are due to the alcohol content of this beverage; however, Damiana was listed in the National Formulary from 1888–1947 and was recommended by physicians for menstrual difficulties including headache linked to monthly cycles, acne, insufficient flow, delayed menstruation in adolescent girls, irritability and nervousness, and lack of sexual desire.

Dosages

Tea	1 tsp crushed or powdered leaf to 1 cup water, steeped for 10–15minutes; 2–3 cups/day
Tincture/Extract	10–20 drops 3×/day
Capsules	300–500 mg 3×/day

Caution

No cautions have been noted for the use of this herb except a slight laxative effect.

Dandelion (Taraxacum officionale)

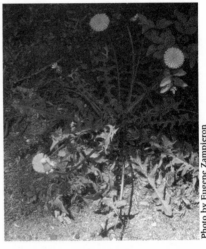

Almost everyone can recognize a dandelion plant, which grows in many areas all over the world. It is used as food and medicine by cultures everywhere. If you are interested in starting to do some wildcrafting, consider collecting dandelion since it is nontoxic and so easy to recognize. The inner strength of this plant is reflected by the amount of time, energy, and money people spend trying to eradicate it from their suburban lawns! Its strength and tenacity is quite apparent. The name "Dandelion" is derived from French , and translates to *tooth of the lion,* referring to the serrated edges of the leaves. Dandelion is a storehouse of nutrients, containing proteins, carotenoids, and minerals which all help to build and cleanse the liver.

The liver is intimately related to all female health problems involving the metabolism of hormones. If the liver is working well, it will break down aggressive estrogen into less harmful varieties, leading to fewer PMS symptoms such as breast tenderness, headaches, and acne. If the liver is working too hard due to the presence of an overload of toxins from poor diet, stress, and other factors, it will not be able to effectively break down estrogen. Also, the same factors, such as xenoestrogens found in commercially

107

raised meat, that cause the liver to be overburdened, also raises the levels of aggressive estrogens. This high aggressive estrogen level is a major cause of PMS, infertility, fibrocystic breasts and ovaries, endometriosis, and difficult menopause symptoms. The liver also actually forms some hormones such as small amounts of testosterone in women. Dandelion, along with other liver protective and cleansing herbs such as burdock and milk thistle, can help clear the liver of toxins and increase its ability to break down estrogen.

Gathering Your Own Dandelions

Find a lawn or field with dandelion that has not been sprayed with toxic chemicals. Bring along a long screwdriver, paper bag, and small shovel. Find the place where the dandelion plant is attached to the ground. Insert the screwdriver at the base of the plant and rotate it all around until the entire plant is loosened. Use the small shovel to loosen the plant even more. Its best to get as much of the root as possible. Shake off loose dirt and place the whole plant in the paper bag.

Every part of the dandelion is edible. Make tea by placing the whole plant, leaves, flowers, and roots in a pot and cover with water. Bring to a simmer for 5 minutes. Cool and drink. The leaves can be added to salad. They are better fresh in the early spring because they get rather bitter as they age. The plant can be dried and saved for later use . Dandelion is available in health food stores as extracts and capsules.

Dosages	
Tea	1 tsp herb or root to 1 cup water 3 cups/day
Tincture/Extract	20 ml 3×/day
Capsules	2 (500 mg) caps 2×/day

Caution

None known; avoid use with acute gall bladder illness.

Dong Quai (Angelica sinensis)

Dong quai is the medicinal root of a species of the *Angelica* plant genus. The plant has the umbrella shaped flower top that is characteristic of the *Umbelliferae* family. The medicinal part is the root; yellow to brown on the outside and white on the inside. Dong quai grows in China, where it has been used medicinally, especially in formulas for women, for thousand of years. The plant can grow in temperate climates worldwide. Plant some in your garden and you will experience the power of Dong quai—the plant itself gets large strong leaves and has a warm dark green color. It is called by several names in herbal literature including dong guai, dang gui, tang kuei, and tang twei.

Scientific research performed on extracts of Dong quai supports its ancient folkloric uses. Pharmacological effects include analgesic activity along with a powerful ability to relax smooth muscle. Dong quai can help reduce high blood pressure, ease asthma, and relax the coronary arteries. Many classical and patent Chinese remedies for blood pressure, migraine headaches, asthma, and angina chest pains contain this herb. Dong quai contains ferulic acid, which acts as an anticoagulant on blood cells, making them less "sticky," and also has an analgesic effect. Ligustilide is a chemical component of this plant which may explain its antispasmotic effect that aids menstrual cramps, headaches,

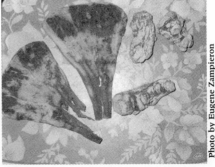

Photo by Eugene Zampieron

109

and also acts to tone the uterus. Dong quai contains vitamins A, E, and B-12—which may be one component in its documented effects increasing red blood cell counts in anemia sufferers—as well as folic acid. It also contains various essential oils and bioflavonoids.

Dong quai can be a woman's best friend. It is recognized as a particulary useful herb in natural health care for women. It relieves common imbalances such as PMS (bloating, mood swings, muscle aches), menstrual cramps, infertility, and menopausal vaginal dryness. Dong quai has tonic properties that help increase energy and vitality. It also increases peripheral circulation and is a mild sedative and antispasmotic. Dong quai can aid during labor by increasing uterine contractions. The name "Dong quai" translates to "proper order" because it balances the entire female system.

Dong quai is used as a dry root, sliced. In Chinese medicine it is usually part of a formula added to nutritious soups.

FOUR THINGS SOUP

Handful of Dong quai
Handful of peony
Handful of rehmannia
Handful of ligusticum
2 quarts water

A special tea called Four Things Soup contains dong quai, peony, rehmannia, and ligusticum. All of these ingredients can be found in a Chinese apothecary (see Resources, page 185). Add one handful of each herb to two quarts water and simmer for one hour.

Dong quai is the main ingredient in the Chinese patent medicine *Women's Eight Treasure Pills,* also called *Precious Pills.* Dong quai is standardized to 8,000 to 11,000 ppm of ligustilide by some herbal manufacturers.

Dosages

Four Things Soup	2–3 cups per day
Patent Medicines	4 pellets, 3×/day, use from day 7 to day 21 of menstrual cycle
Standardized Extract	10 drops 3×/day
Capsules	200 mg 3×/day

Cautions

- Do not use in early pregnancy.
- May cause heavy bleeding.
- Discontinue use during menstruation.
- If used while going through menopause, Dong quai may restart the period even if you have not had a period in over a year. This is not dangerous but may cause concern.
- Dong quai has been noted to increase photosensitivity on rare occasions.

False Unicorn Root (Chamaelirium luteum, Veratrum luteum)

False unicorn is a member of the lily family and grows in low moist ground along the Mississippi delta. It was used by Native Americans in this region to promote health in women. The plant is becoming rare in the wild, but is being cultivated for use as a medicinal herb. For this reason herbalists suggest that you choose a cultivated instead of a wildcrafted product. False unicorn is known by several other names including helonias, starwort, blazing star, and fairywand. The star names refer to the plant's beautiful white star-like flowers that appear in May and June. They grow on long stalks (fairywands) that were thought to look like unicorn's horns. Another name is "devil's bite," which it earned by having roots—the medicinal part of the plant—that look like someone gnawed on them. Supposedly the devil was not happy with the healing effects this plant afforded women!

False unicorn contains steroidal saponins (chamaelirin) which may be responsible for its toning effects on the uterus. Although there have been no major scientific studies to date on this herb, folkloric use has focused on its ability to increase fertility and to avoid miscarriage, especially if a women experiences a "pulling down feeling." It is also useful for strengthening the kidney and liver, and has diuretic properties.

Dosages

Tea	1 tsp herb to 1 cup water, 3 cups/day
Extract	10 drops, 2×/day
Capsules	2 caps (200 mg) 1–2×/day

Cautions

In higher doses , nausea and vomiting may occur in sensitive individuals.

Fenugreek
(Trigonella Foenum-Graceum)

Fenugreek has been recognized as a medicinal plant for centuries. The Egyptians, Greeks, and Romans used it for medicine and as a spice. The annual herbaceous plant grows in the Mediterranean, India, Morocco, Egypt, and England and has yellow-white flowers in the summer. The aromatic seeds are the medicinal part used. They are often roasted, ground, and used to flavor curry. Powdered seeds mixed with water or oil make a soothing paste that can be used as a skin emollient, useful for inflamed swellings or rashes on the skin. Taken internally, fenugreek is used to treat bronchitis, coughs, respiratory problems, and sinus conditions especially if due to allergies. Fenugreek tea, capsules, or tincture helps to stabilize blood sugar, increases milk supply during breastfeeding, and is considered an aphrodisiac. Fenugreek can increase a nursing mother's milk within one to three days. Once an adequate level of milk production is reached fenugreek can be discontinued. The aromatic compounds in the fenugreek seeds have a maple-syrup-like odor.

Dosages	
Tea	½ tsp seed to 1 cup water, steeped 5 minutes, 1–3 cups/day
Tincture/Extract	10 drops 2×/day
Capsules	500 mg 2×/day
Poultice	Soak ground seeds in enough hot water to make a paste, mix with oil, and apply to skin.

Caution

The urine of mother and child may start to have a maple syrup odor, potentially leading to a misdiagnosis of maple syrup urine disease. Be sure to tell your health care practitioner if you are using fenugreek while nursing. May increase the effects of drugs used for diabetes.

CYCLES OF LIFE

Ginger (Zingiber officinale)

The name ginger is derived from the Indian Sanskrit word *singagera* which means "grows like a horn." The fresh ginger root definitely does fit that description. Indonesia grows the largest ginger supply in the world, but it is also found in India, Jamaica, China, and throughout tropical Asian countries. Ginger is commonly used as a culinary spice.

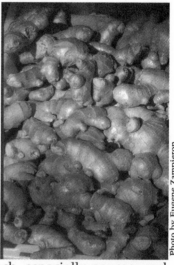

Photo by Eugene Zampieron

In traditional Chinese medicine ginger root is one of the most frequently prescribed herbs, along with ginseng, astragalus, and licorice root. It is used for coughs, colds, upset stomach, especially nausea, and circulation. Chinese medicine describes ginger as a warming herb which increases the flow of chi (life force energy) as well as the movement of stagnant blood and lymphatic fluid. Ginger is an excellent remedy for pain and has been shown to have similar action to aspirin, blocking substances such as prostaglandins and leukotrienes, which are involved with inflammation. Ginger has been scientifically studied for its effects on nausea and was found to work as well as the drug Dramamine, without any side effects. Ginger can be used during pregnancy for morning sickness. It also contains zingibain, an enzyme that dissolves plaque and blood clots. This enzyme decreases high blood levels of cholesterol, artherosclerosis, strokes, heart attacks and high blood pressure. Ginger has a high level of antioxidant activity, protecting the body from damage due to free radicals. Ginger can also stimulate white blood cells to engulf bacteria and other pathogens. It helps kill many kinds of disease causing microorganisms.

Ginger is also excellent to use externally as a compress. The ginger compress will increase circulation to the area and bring welcome pain relief. The ginger compress can be used after childbirth directly on the perineum to help heal and decrease swelling, or on any painful joint or muscle.

GINGER TEA—WARMING DIGESTIVE AID

    1 3-inch ginger root, sliced thin
    1 tsp cloves
    1 Tbs green cardamom pods
    3 cinnamon sticks

Add all ingredients to 2 quarts water. Simmer for 10 minutes. Drink 1 to 3 cups a day. Can be rewarmed or used as iced tea.

GINGER COMPRESS

    1 3 to 6-inch ginger root, grated or finely chopped
    1 Tbs fenugreek seeds
    1 Tbs dried comfrey

Add all ingredients to 1 quart water, Simmer for 5 minutes. Allow to cool to comfortable temperature. Soak clean washcloth in mixture. Apply to skin area. Cover with a terrycloth towel to keep heat in. Remove when cool. Repeat as needed.

DR. EUGENE ZAMPIERON'S ZINGIBER ZING

    ½- to ¾-inch slice of organic ginger root
    1 organic Granny Smith apple or ½ cup apple juice
    1 cup seltzer or club soda
    2 to 3 drops stevia liquid extract or honey to taste

Juice the ginger root in a juice extractor or grate finely by hand. Juice the apple or pour the apple juice over the ginger. Strain to remove grated ginger and combine with soda. Add stevia or honey to taste. Add ice if desired. Enjoy!

Dosages	
Tea	1–3 cups/day
Tincture/Extract	10 drops 2×/day
Capsules	500 mg 2×/day

Cautions

Although there is no known toxicity, ginger can cause a burning sensation in the mouth or stomach in sensitive individuals if they use too much. If used at the same time as pharmaceutical blood thinners, be sure your physician checks the blood so it does not become too thin. The German Commission E recommends that ginger should not be used during pregnancy, although historically it has been used for the nausea associated with morning sickness in cultures around the world.

Green Beans (Phaseolus vulgaris)

Green beans are one vegetable that has actually become a staple in the standard american diet. Unfortunately, they are often served overcooked and/or canned, which may deplete many of their nutritive factors. Green beans are one of the few members of the vegetable kingdom that actually contain phytoestrogens—estrone, estriol and estradiol—that occur naturally as three forms of estrogen in humans. Green beans have long been heralded in folk traditions as an aid for fertility and other women's health issues. The Doctrine of Signatures of this vegetable is interesting to note. The combination of an elongated phallic shape, along with the coddling of the bean seed within a womb-like structure, unites the male and female aspects of fertility.

HEALTHY GREEN BEANS

Steam fresh green beans for 5 to 8 minutes or until tender. Place in another pan and add olive oil. Warm slightly—do not fry. Add sliced organic almond; season with herbs such as thyme, parsley, garlic, and/or oregano. Toss all together and serve.

CYCLES OF LIFE

Green Foods

"Green foods" is a general term that refers to several different types of plants that are very high in chlorophyll. This includes spirulina, chlorella, and blue-green algae (unicellular water plants); and barley grass and wheat grass, which are juiced and dried. Although each of these green foods have somewhat different properties, they all contain high amounts of chlorophyll, the green pigment in plants. Chlorophyll has a very similar chemical structure to blood except it has a magnesium molecule instead of the iron found in the heme portion of the blood. Chlorophyll is highly nutritious and encourages the growth of healthy tissues leading to clear skin and lustrous hair. It also discourages the growth of disease causing microorganisms. Increasing chlorophyll intake will help to regulate glandular functions and provide vitamins, such as B-6, B-12 (rarely found in the vegetable kingdom), C, K, and folic acid, as well as minerals and amino acids. Green foods are an important dietary supplement that can help in every life cycle. A daily ration of green foods can help to compensate for an otherwise nutrient poor diet, so common in girls going through menarche. Women of any age will notice a calm energy after a few weeks of adding green foods to their daily routine. It is recommended for infertility, to help balance deficiencies that worsen PMS, for extra nutrition during pregnancy and after birth, and for maintaining high level wellness during menopause and beyond.

Grow Your Own

A fun way to include wheat or barley grass in the diet is to grow it yourself. This can even be done as a science project for a biology class. Buy organic winter wheat berries or barley pearls at your health food store. Place about a cup of the seeds in a glass jar and cover with water. Allow the mixture to sit for 36 hours, shaking once or twice during that time. You'll notice little bubbles starting to form in the water indicating that the seeds are ready to plant. Prepare a glass 2 to 3-inch high baking dish filled with a combination of peat moss and top soil. Moisten the soil. Pour the water off the seeds (this water can be used as a drink to help establish friendly bacteria in the intestines. It is also a useful douche for vaginal yeast infections.) Place the soaked seeds on top of the soil—just one layer thick. Use a water spray bottle to moisten the seeds. Spray them once or twice a day to keep the seeds moist. Keep the tray out of the sun for the first few days until you notice red seedlings shooting up—which will turn green in a few more days. Once the green grass starts to grow, keep it in partial sunlight, but don't allow it to dry out. After about a week you can start using the grass. Get a manual or electric juicer to put the grass through, or simply cut the grass and chew it, extracting the green juice and then spitting out the spent grass.

Dosage	
Green Foods	1–2 Tbs/day

He (Ho) Shou Wu
(Polygonum multiflorum)

He Shou Wu (also known as Ho Shou Wu) or most commonly in the United States as *Fo-Ti,* is one of China's premium herbs and is revered for its mysterious properties of rejuvenation and anti-aging. It has been used for over a thousand years as a royal tonic.

He Shou Wu is a vine-like plant with heart shaped leaves that can grow to a length of seven to ten meters! It is related to the common edible North American weeds "lady's thumb" and "smart weed." The medicine referred to as *Radix Polygoni multiflori* is derived from the enormous tuberous reddish brown root. The Chinese *Materia Medica* lists He Shou Wu as an herb that nourishes the blood; cleanses the liver and kidneys; supports the joints, ligaments, tendons, muscles, and sinews; increases the chi (life force) of the liver and kidneys; increases fertility in both women and men; corrects anemia; is helpful in arthritis and chronic fatigue; and has the unique ability to regrow hair and to return grey hair to its natural color. The name He Shou Wu translates to "Mr. He's Black Hair Tonic," or "King He's White Hair Turned Black." Chinese legends describe a sickly, middle-aged, infertile man named He who discovered this herb and reversed the aging process. He fathered many children into old age and turned his gray hair back to jet black. Dr. Eugene Zampieron, N.D., confirmed this effect in several patients who used this herb and effectively reversed their hair from gray back to their natural color. Ho Shou Wu also increases the odds of conception in infertile women.

Ho Shou Wu is available in Chinese apothecaries as Shou Wu Pian, Shou Wu Zhi, or Zhong Guo Shou Wu Zhi.

Dosage	
Pills	5–10 pills, 3×/ day

Cautions

May have a slight laxative effect.

Horse Chestnut
(Aesculus hippocastanum)

The horse chestnut is the seed formed by a large tree that is grows in Asia, southeastern Europe, and the northeastern United States. The leaves of this majestic tree are quite distinctive and look like a large hand with five to seven fingers.

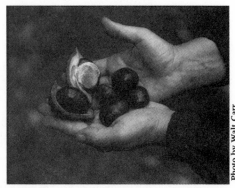

Photo by Walt Carr

Horse chestnut was used as a food and medicine for horses by the Turks. They used it as a specific remedy for horses with a condition called broken wind and other respiratory ailments with coughing and fever. It was also pulverized and wrapped around horses legs as a poultice for sore joints and skin conditions. By the 1740s, the horse chestnut tree was introduced into Europe and America as an ornamental garden tree. Shortly thereafter, Native Americans began to use the nuts or seeds produced in the fall. They were crushed, prepared into a topical salve, and used for tired legs and hemorrhoids. The Eclectic physicians at the turn of the century used horse chestnut extract for leg throbbing and varicose veins.

Modern day science collaborates folk medicine's use of horse chestnut. The extract has been widely researched, especially in Germany, where it is used for chronic circulatory problems including varicose veins, hemorrhoids, and leg swelling. Scientific studies have shown its effectiveness for these purposes.[16]

Horse chestnut contains several active ingredients. They are a complex grouping of compounds called *escin*, which strengthen the structure, function, and tone of veins. This helps swelling, pain, and unsightly varicose veins.

CYCLES OF LIFE

Gathering Your Own Horse Chestnuts

Don't confuse this tree with sweet chestnut. Consult your local herbalist or a plant guidebook. Once you learn to recognize horse chestnut it is an easy tree to identify. Horse chestnut trees have a strong personality. This may be experienced as a powerful energy field. The flowers are beautiful white torches in the spring, followed by hand-like leaves. In the fall, the tree will be covered with pods that have spiny projections. After the pods fall to the ground, they split open to reveal the beautiful seed or fruit of the horse chestnut. I find these seeds absolutely beautiful. They have a smooth, rich mahogany tone. I gather them just to hold them as a stress reducing aid! After my pockets are filled with all the seed friends I can carry, I then fill up large zip-lock baggies with lots of seeds and store them in the freezer where they can last at least two years.

VARICOSE VEIN HORSE CHESTNUT POULTICE

3 or 4 horse chestnuts
Handful of calendula or marigold blossoms
1 cup olive oil
1 Tbs witch hazel
Thickening agent (see below)

Place the horse chestnuts in a pan, and cover with water. Bring to a boil, simmer for a few minutes to soften. Smash up the chestnuts. Add the blossoms and olive oil. Bring mixture to a simmer for 10 minutes. Do not boil. Stir all together. Add the witch hazel. Now add a thickening agent—this can be flour, corn meal, agar, or anything else that holds the mixture together.

Smooth the herb mixture on affected areas, such as varicose veins. Wrap with gauze. (Cloth diapers covered with plastic to avoid leakage work well.) Leave in place several hours.

Dosages	
Tea	1 tsp crushed seed to 1 cup water, steeped 5-10 min. 3 cups/day
Extract/Tincture	1–2 ml 3×/day
Capsules	1 cap (250–500 mg) 2×/day

Horse chestnut is often combined with other herbs that are helpful for circulation (*e.g.*, gotu kola, gingko biloba, butcher's broom). It is generally standardized to 16–20% triterpene glycosides.

Cautions

Some people experience gastrointestinal upset, nausea, headache, or skin rash. Use a small amount at first and gauge your reaction.

CYCLES OF LIFE

Jamaican Dogwood (Piscidia spp.)

Jamaican dogwood is a giant member of the pea family and is a powerful herb for pain. The tree grows in Jamaica, the Bahamas, Mexico, southern Texas, and Florida. The bark is used as the medicinal component. It is peeled off the outer layer of the root or the tree branches. The Arawak Indians, the original inhabitants of the Caribbean, used it as a fishing aid. They would beat the root or bark into a mash, dam up the stream, and spread the dogwood into the water. The fish would become lethargic and float to the surface. It was then "easy spearing" for the Arawaks!

In the Maroon culture, Jamaican dogwood is used by the bush doctors for nerve pain such as sciatica, toothaches, and migraines. A poultice of the root is tied around sprains as a potent anti-inflammatory. It was also used as a sedative for hysteria, insomnia, and anxiety. As an antispasmodic, it can ease painful cramping of all muscles, but especially targets those of the uterus. This makes it especially helpful for women's health issues, including labor pains and severe menstrual cramping.

Its active principles contain glycosides including *piscidin* and *jamaicin*; it also contains bioflavonoid glycosides.

Dosages

Tea	The bark can be made into a strong decoction; 1 tsp bark in 1 cup water, steeped for 10 min.
Extracts/Tinctures	10 drops 2×/day
Capsules	Not widely available. *BotanoDyne* (see www.naturesanswer.com) combines Jamaican dogwood with kava kava root, white willow bark, and other herbs.
Solid Extract	¼ teaspoon is equivalent to approx. 8,000 mg; use ¼ tsp every hour for severe cramping and pain until relieved.

Cautions

- Do not use in early pregnancy.
- Do not use for the first time while operating heavy machinery or while driving until you know if it makes you feel sleepy.

Kava Kava (Piper methysticum)

Kava kava grows in the South Pacific islands and in Hawaii. It is a wide-leafed vine, a relative to the pepper plant. The part of the plant used to make the medicinal extract is the large root or rhizome. It has been used for thousands of years. Captain Cook described its use in 1768 during one of his 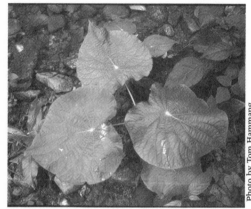 South Sea voyages. Traditional use of kava involves pounding the fresh root into a pulp, and then cooking it into a thick tea or soup. It is often served in a coconut shell. The kava drink tastes bitter and causes a tingling sensation on the tongue and throat. Kava is used to relax the body and mind, to produce a tranquil state, to enhance sociability and friendliness, and to ease pain. It can be helpful for arthritis, fibromyalgia, PMS, menstrual cramps, labor, and postpartum pain. It is touted as an aphrodisiac for women, although it may produce enough muscular relaxation to interfere with an erection in men. The most common use of kava in western medicine is as an antianxiety agent.[17] The active ingredients in kava include kava lactones. It is available in health food stores as a prepared extract or capsule, and may be standardized to contain 30–50% kava lactones.

Photo by Tom Hammang

Dosages	
Tea	2–3 cups
Extract	20 drops
Capsules	100 mg

Cautions

- High doses of Kava over extended periods of time can cause a rough skin condition called Kava dermatitis. It is reversible if Kava is discontinued.
- Kava can change the way you feel.
- When first using Kava do not drive or operate heavy machinery. Try it first in the evening or when all the day's responsibilities are over.

Licorice Root (Glycyrrhiza glabra)

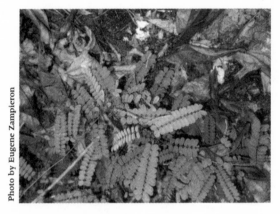

Photo by Eugene Zampieron

The word "licorice" is often associated with a distinctive flavor. The truth is most licorice flavored condiments in the United States are actually made from anise or fennel. In Europe, however, true licorice is often used. Linnaeus coined the term *glycyrrhiza* from *glykys* , meaning sweet, and *rhiza,* or root. Glycyrrhizin is fifty times sweeter than sugar. It is often added to herbal tea mixtures that contain bitter herbs such as dandelion. The sweet flavor of the licorice covers the bitterness and adds to the medicinal value.

Licorice root is one of the most widely studied herbal medicines. It has been proven to help block viral reproduction,[18] and is used by physicians knowledgeable in herbal medicine for herpes, HIV, and hepatitis. It is effective against *Streptococcus mutants,* a major cause of dental cavities. In Britain, licorice is the main ingredient in prescription drugs such as Caved-S, and Carbenoloxone, used for peptic ulcers.

DGL refers to deglycyrrhized licorice, which is specifically used for stomach ulcers and canker sores. This form avoids the possible side-effect of high blood pressure from the glycyrrhizin naturally found in licorice. In Japan, the intravenous prescription drug made from licorice, Stronger Neominophagan-C, is used to protect the liver from toxic damage and to kill hepatitis virus.

Licorice is a useful herb for female problems such as PMS and menopause. It contains specific compounds that have been documented to have estrogenic-like properties.[19] These phytoestrogens can help balance negative effects caused by more aggressive estrogens by fitting into receptor sites and blocking the uptake of aggressive estrogens. Licorice can act as a true adaptogen, increasing or decreasing the amount of estrogen in the body depending on a woman's needs. Licorice is an effective anti-inflammatory, and has the ability to block a particular enzyme that breaks down the body's natural cortisone.

Dosages	
Topically	For cold or canker sores, use as needed
Tea	Add 3-4 inches of licorice root to 1 qt water, simmered for 5 min
Tincture/Extract	1–2 ml 2×/day, usually combined with other herbs
Capsules	100–500 mg 1–2×/day
DGL tablets	(standardized to 1.5% glycyrrhizin) chew and mix well with saliva. Take two 380mg 20 minutes before eating

Cautions

Licorice root can have side effects due to the glycyrrhetic acid which can decrease potassium levels and increase sodium, leading to water retention and an increase in blood pressure. However, after thousands of years of the use of licorice root in many Chinese patent medicines, there are no reported problems of this type when small amounts are used in herbal mixtures. The DGL form does not raise blood pressure. Do not combine with Furosemide/Thiazide diuretics, digitalis, or other antiarrythmic medications. Check with your health care provider if you are on any prescription medications.

Milk Thistle (Silybum marianum)

Milk thistle grows in the wild throughout Europe and North America. It has large purple flowers surrounded by a sharp array of thorns, hence the name "thistle." Legend has it that milk from Mother Mary runs through the veins of the plant's leaves. In fact, milk thistle is an excellent galactogogue (increases lactation). The leaves can be eaten once the spiny stickers are removed; the taste is similar to an artichoke. The ripe seeds (actually tiny fruits) are gathered in late fall to extract the highly medicinal components.

Milk thistle is used first and foremost for its protective and regenerative effect on the liver. Scientific studies have shown that milk thistle has two distinct actions on liver cells—it changes the structure of the outer membranes of the cells so that toxins cannot enter and increases ribosomal proteins that helps the liver regenerate new cells. Milk thistle is a useful herb to help in all situations where liver detoxification is indicated. In relation to women's health issues, it is especially helpful for all imbalances linked to excessive estrogen including PMS, cystic breasts, fibroids, endometriosis, and infertility (since an overburdened liver cannot break down excessive estrogen). It is also useful for acne, psoriasis, other skin conditions; and all alcohol, drug, or chemically induced liver damage including hepatitis, cirrhosis, and Tylenol (acetaminophen) toxicity. Believe it or not, milk thistle has antioxidant activity that is a thousand times greater than vitamin E!

Milk thistle has no known side effects, so it is prudent to take it as a preventive measure if you are involved in a toxic work environment such as that of cosmetologists, painters, construction personnel, print shop workers, artists, and dry cleaners, or if you indulge in social alcohol drinking or recreational drug use. It will also help to protect the liver from damage due to prescription drugs.

Dosages	
Tea	1 Tbs finely ground seeds and leaf powder to 1 cup water
Tincture/Extract	1–2 ml 2×/day
Capsules	200 mg 3×/day

Milk thistle is often standardized to 75-80% silymarin.

Motherwort (Leonurus cardiaca)

Motherwort is a perennial member of the mint family, identified by a square stem. Ancient Greek botanists thought that the leaves resembled the tail of the lion, and named it *Leonurus*. *Cardiaca*, refers to its tonic effects for the heart. Motherwort means "elder woman" and "plant."

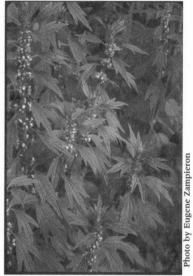

Photo by Eugene Zampieron

There are many legends about motherwort. One story from China tells of a young boy who was banished from his village due to a minor crime. He moved to a valley where the water supply flowed through an abundant field of motherwort. He drank this water daily and was reported to live three centuries.

Motherwort was traditionally used to alleviate headaches, painful periods, nervous irritability, and menopausal symptoms, especially:

- Insomnia and anxiety
- Palpitations of the heart, especially from 2 to 4 A.M.
- Mental and emotional agitation
- Hot flashes

Motherwort acts as a bitter which helps digestion and assimilation of nutrients. It relaxes the smooth muscles of the body, resulting in lower blood pressure, and has also been used in combination with other herbs like skullcap (*Scutellaria spp.*) for the control of seizures.

In Chinese traditional medicine it is called Yi Mu Cao, or "benefit mother herb," and is believed to specifically influence the heart and liver acupuncture meridians. The Chinese felt it invigorated and moved blood and chi and helped to regulate the menstrual cycle.

The chemical compounds in Motherwort include iridoid glycosides, diterpenes, and flavonoids which may scientifically explain its calming effect on the heart, mind, and spirit.

Dosages

Tea	½ tsp dried herb to 1 cup water
Extract/Tincture	2 ml 2×/day
Capsules	200-300 mg, 3×/ day

Cautions

- Since motherwort can increase menstrual flow, avoid using it if heavy bleeding is a problem.
- Do not use in pregnancy.

CYCLES OF LIFE

Nettle (Urtica dioica)

If you have ever brushed up against a stinging nettle plant you understand why it is called "stinging." The tiny hairs that cover the stem and leaves of the plant are stingers coated with a chemical that burns the skin for about half an hour. The stingers contain formic acid, histamine, serotonin, and acetylcholine, which irritate the skin and cause the itching and burning. Notice the latin name of this plant—*Urtica*. In medical terminology, *uticaria* means hives—the little welts caused by the stinging nettle is just like a hive. The leaves and stems of the nettle, once the stingers have been removed by boiling or freezing , are used medicinally. They contain flavonoids including rutin which may help to explain nettle's use for allergic reactions. Nettle is highly nutrious and contains minerals (especially potassium), vitamin C, protein, and other nourishing factors. Nettle can be used as a tonic, especially helpful for kidney and urinary ailments. It also can aid with fatigue, headaches, and other aches and pains; and ease the transition of the hormonal storms of menarche, PMS, and menopause. Perhaps the sting is a wake-up call to the endocrine system. Nettle can help increase the robustness of young girls and older women who are fragile and pale, helps the body generate strong blood, and reverses anemia. It is a good tonic herb that can be used daily to increase overall nutritional status.

Gathering Your Own Nettle

If you choose to pick your own nettle use the following technique to avoid getting stung. The best time to pick nettle is while it is flowering, although it can be gathered during any time of the year while it is growing. The leaves and ariel parts of the plants, as well as the roots, are used medicinally. Bring a paper bag along with a large tweezer, scissors, and heavy gardening gloves. Use the tweezers to select the leaf stalk that you want, and guide it into the paper bag. Then cut it at the base and shake it down into the bag. The stingers are dissolved when the nettle is made into a tea or placed directly into the freezer. The frozen nettle can then be used at a future time. Of course, you may choose to skip the stinging excitement of field collection and get your already stingless nettle tea, extract or capsules at a health food store.

Dosages	
Tea	1 tsp leaf to 1 cup water, 2–4 cups/day
Tincture/extract	2 ml 2×/day
Capsules	2 500 mg caps 2×/day

Oats (Avena sativa)

The oat plant is a tall hollow grass with round seeds on the top of the stalk that is the commonly used oat. The plants mature in late summer, but just before that, the seeds are in a semi-solid milky state. This is the best stage to collect the seeds for making extracts or tinctures. Every part of the plant is useful: oat groats are the unprocessed seeds; oatmeal is the seeds after they have been rolled or ground; oatbran is the husks from the seeds; amd oat straw is the plant's dried stalk.

Oats are extremely high in nutrition, and can be added to the diet regularly to maintain health. People sensitive to gluten may experience a cross-sensitivity with the use of oats as a cereal, but can use it as a tincture/extract. Oats contain proteins; minerals; sterols, including beta-sitosterol; beta-glucans, which enhance immune function; vitamin B-complex; vitamin E; and fiber. The high fiber content has been touted by conventional medicine and mainstream advertising alike to be cancer-protective.

Oats provide nerve food which offsets the effects of stress. It is helpful for depression, anxiety, reduced sex drive, fatigue, and convalescing from illness or childbirth. Oats are also part of a heart healthy program when reduction of blood cholesterol is desired. Their high nutrient content helps the body form hormones efficiently by supporting the thyroid, adrenal, uterus, and ovaries; and the testicles in men. The saying "sowing your wild oats" refers to the use of oats to increase sexual function. When oats are soaked, they release a white-milky fluid which mirrors the appearance of sexual fluids.

Oats are also useful externally on the skin for itching, rashes, and improvement of the complexion.

OATMEAL SMOOTHY FACIAL

¼ cup oatmeal
1 cup aloe vera juice
A few drops jojoba oil
A few drops lavender oil

Mix together all ingredients and allow to stand for five minutes. Add a few tablespoons of hot water to create a smooth paste. Apply to face. Leave on for up to 15 minutes. Rinse off.

Dosages

Oatmeal	a bowl a day (choose organic oats if possible)
Tincture/Extract	10–20 ml 2×/day
Capsules	500–1000 mg 2×/day
Bath	Heat 1 qt of water with 1 cup of oats or a handful of oatstraw. Strain; add liquid to bathwater.

Red Clover (Trifolium pratense)

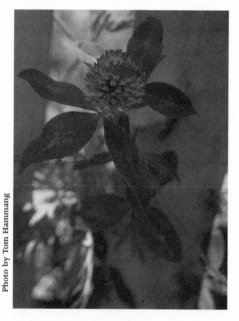

Photo by Tom Hammang

The red clover flower grows in many areas of the world including Europe and temperate regions in the U.S. This herb is easily recognized. It is similar to the more common white clover that grows on lawns, much to the suburban gardener's dismay, but the herbalist's delight! The red clover is about twelve inches high, and sports the distinctive red flower top. Many would refer to this color as purple, thus the other common name of this plant, purple clover. It is also called cow grass because it was grown as cattle fodder as early as 1747.[20]

Red Clover has been used as a medicine in all parts of the world. Traditional Chinese medicine recommended its use in herbal combinations for coughs and other respiratory ailments. It is part of the well-known anticancer Hoxey formula, which combines red clover with burdock, licorice root, and other herbs. In the 1890s the pharmaceutical company Parke-Davis marketed red clover for its antispasmotic and antimucus effects for obstructive coughs, especially whooping cough, as well as for its mild sedative actions. Common uses included antispasmotic, expectorant, skin healing, and blood-cleansing action.

Although old time remedies did not focus on this herb for its female balancing properties, modern research has revealed that the chemical constituents contained in red clover include glycosides and isoflavones, in particular genistein, biochanin-A, and diadzein. These estrogenic-like compounds can help balance the female system and are cancer protective.

A fascinating aspect of the Doctrine of Signature principle and this plant's use, particularly for adolescent girls, is the botanical description of its leaflets as pubescent (covered with soft hair-like fuzz), which mirrors an obvious characteristic of puberty. Interesting, too, is the ovate-pod shape of the fruit. We often see this in estrogen-containing plants such as green beans and soy.

Pick Your Own

Pick red clover yourself in a vacant lot or field. Simply pop off the red flower tops. Use some fresh and dry the rest by placing them in a paper bag. Keep in a cool dry place. If they get moldy, throw them away. Use as a tea or skin wash, for acne or other skin problems. Red clover is also available commercially as an extract and capsules.

Dosages	
Tea	1 Tbs flower tops, fresh or dried, in 1 cup boiled water 2–3 cups/day
Extract/Tincture	10 drops 3×/day
Capsules	2 (250 mg) caps 3×/day

Red Raspberry (Rubus idaeus)

Red raspberries grow in dense thickets on a prolific, red prickly vine. It is a member of the rose family and is comfortable growing deep in the woods or in backyards. Raspberries are a delicious fruit beloved to wildlife and humans alike. They are full of nutritious vitamins and minerals such as vitamin C, carotenes, niacin, thiamine, calcium, and magnesium; and are a great source of antioxidants. The leaf of the vine is the part that is most often used as herbal medicine. It has been dubbed the "vine of female vitality." This claim is backed by scientific research. The medical journal *Lancet* published a study in 1941 describing the normalizing effect that red raspberry leaf extract has on the uterus. If the smooth muscle of the uterus was in spasm the extract caused it to relax; if the muscle was flaccid the extract caused it to contract.

Red Raspberry is one herb that is considered safe to use during pregnancy. It is also perfect to use as a preparatory for pregnancy and to aid in fertility. As one might suspect through the Doctrine of Signatures, the prolific nature of the growth of the vine signals

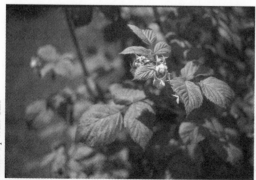

Photo by Walt Carr

its use for increasing fertility in both men and women. It helps to reduce the nausea of morning sickness (add ginger to the mixture for greater relief of this symptom). Midwives and herbalists claim that it also helps to tone the ligaments of the uterus to ease childbith, reduces hemorrhage after birth, and enriches colostrum, the immune-stimulating first milk of nursing mothers.

During labor, red raspberry tea can be sipped, or made into ice cubes and sucked. It can help promote regular contractions. Prepare a poultice of the leaves and apply over the uterus to decrease menstrual cramps or to help a prolapsed uterus. The effectiveness of this poultice is due to the herbs astringent effect. This astringent nature also help's with spider veins and mouth ulcers.

Pick Your Own

Find some vines deep in the woods where they have not been sprayed with toxic pesticides or grow them in your own backyard. Pick the berries when they are ripe. Store any that you do not eat in the freezer. They can be added to fresh veggie juice or used for pancakes or in baked goods all year long. Pick the leaves after the berries are gone in midsummer to late fall. Dry the leaves by laying them flat, not touching each other, in a dry area out of the sun. After drying keep them in a sealable baggie or glass jar. Remember to label them since dried herbs can resemble each other.

Dosages	
Tea	Add 3 fresh leaves or 1 Tbs of dried powdered leaf to 1 cup water, steeped 5-10 min.
Tincture/Extract	1–2 ml 3×/day
Capsules	300-500 mg 2-3×/day

Rose Buds (Rosa spp.)

The rosebud is one of my favorite symbols because my grandmother's nickname for me was Rosebud. The tightly closed rosebud, ready to burst open and become a fully mature flower, is a beautiful mirror image in nature of a young women as she blossoms into womanhood. Roses have a close association to emotional and spiritual expressions throughout history. They are a popular gift that represents love and romance. The rosary beads used in the Catholic religion to count prayers, were originally made from rose petals that were boiled down and rolled into beads. Then, as they were used, they would continue to give off a delightful fragrance.

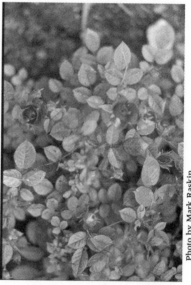

Photo by Mark Raskin

Rosebuds are highly nutritious, containing bioflavonoids and vitamin C, although not as high in this nutrient as rose hips, the fruit of the rosebush. Rose petal tea has a long history of use for mild menstrual cramps, headaches, dizziness, and a weakened constitution. In Chinese medicine, rosebuds are combined with Siberian ginseng for mild depression and to ensure a more joyful mood.

Picking Your Own

Gather rosebuds from rosebushes in your yard or in the wild, as long as they have *not* been sprayed with toxic pesticides. They can be used fresh or dried. To dry them, place the rosebuds on a paper towel in a cool, dry area out of the sun. After drying, keep them in a tightly closed jar. If the flowers become moldy, they are no longer useful.

ROSE PETAL BEADS

Gather rose petals when they are at their brightest phase. Darker colors such as red and lavender colored rose petals hold their color better than yellow petals, which tend to fade. It takes about two handfuls of rose petals to make one bead.

The process of making rose beads is very similar to making apple sauce. Use about 4 cups of rose petals for ten or more beads. One cup of rose petals is approximately 15 petals.

Start by mashing the petals with a fork or in a blender. In a small saucepan, place petals, a small amount of water, and any essential oils such as rose or lavender to enhance bead fragrance. Use enough water to keep the petals from burning. Cover and simmer; stir occasionally for about 1 to 1½ hours. Continue adding water to prevent over-evaporation. Once the mixture forms a thick paste, remove from heat. Allow it to cool to touch. Then take a teaspoon to tablespoon-sized balls of the mixture, depending on the size of the bead you wish to make, and roll it flat with a rolling pin, jar, or candle. Wrap the ends together into a bead shape and let cool on wax paper. After a day, the bead will harden and can be strung.

—Alexandra Porter

SIBERIAN GINSENG & ROSEBUD TEA

This brew immediately lifts the spirits. It can even help overcome a broken heart. Use bulk Siberian ginseng (*Eleutherococcus senticosus*) or prepared tea bags available at a health food store. Use rosebuds you collect yourself, or purchase dried from Chinese herb apothecaries. Use about 1 teaspoon of each herb and cover with 1 cup of boiled water. Allow to steep for 5 to 8 minutes. Add stevia or honey as a sweetener if desired.

Dosages	
Tea	1–3 cups of Siberian ginseng & rosebud tea as needed

Rue (Ruta graveolens)

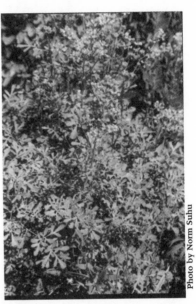

Photo by Norm Suhu

Rue grows prolifically in Italy, the Balkans, and the southern Alps. In the United States it is cultivated as a hardy perennial garden plant. The rue plant has a long history of use in folklore. The club-shaped leaves are the model for the suit of clubs in playing cards. Many believe that if rue is planted by the front door to a home it will keep out negative energy, so it was often called the "heb of grace." The strong pungent odor released from the leaves and stems probably initiated this belief. The dried leaves keep insects away . Both Michaelangelo and Leonardo da Vinci are said to have used a rue leaf tea eyewash for eye fatigue. The homeopathic remedy *Ruta graveolens* used for bruising and rheumatic complaints is made from this plant. The tea has been used as a contraceptive and anti-fertility agent, but can be toxic.

Dosage

Do not use internally.

Caution

Toxic side effects have been reported, including nausea, dizziness, and photosensitivity. The oil on the leaves can cause skin irritation. Never take during pregnancy.

Saint John's Wort
(Hypericum perforatum)

St. John's wort is a herbaceous plant that grows in open fields and waste areas. It is widely distributed in Europe, North and South America, Asia, and Australia. The flowers are used as the medicinal part, and are ready to harvest close to St. John's

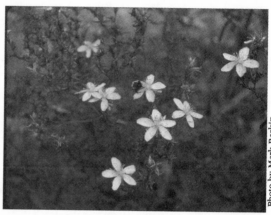

Photo by Mark Raskin

Day—June 24 in England. When harvesting your own, check the edges of the yellow flowers with a magnifying glass for tiny black dots, which contain some of the desired active constituents. Varieties lacking black dots may not be useful as medicine. The species name *perforatum* describes the tiny perforation-like holes that can be seen through the leaves if they are held up to the sunlight. When the bright yellow flowers of St. John's wort are crushed they exude a bright red liquid. This was thought to represent the beheading of St. John the Baptist. This plant is also known as St. Joan's wort.

St. John's wort has been used throughout recorded history. In ancient Greece it was considered an excellent remedy for menstrual cramps, wound healing, headaches, sciatic and nerve pain. It was also hung above the doorway to dispel evil spirits. During the Crusades, the Knights of St. John treated battle wounds with crushed flowers and stems. Modern scientific investigations have confirmed the herb's usefulness for viral infections. In German studies the intravenous drug Hyperforate, extracted from St. John's wort, was shown to inhibit viral replication.

St. John's wort is most well known in the U.S. for its activity as an antidepressant for mild to moderate depression. Several widely accepted scientific studies have shown that it works as well as many prescription antidepressants with fewer side effects.[21] Scientists are still debating exactly how St. John's wort works as an antidepressant. It appears that several mechanisms occur simultaneously. It probably has effects of MAO inhibition. This means it stops the action of the enzyme monoamine oxidase, which breaks down mood-elevating neurotransmitters. This leads to higher levels of these mood elevators which allays depression. St. John's wort also enhances the brain's uptake of GABA (gaba amino butyric acid), a calming and mood elevating amino acid. It may also function as a serotonin reuptake inhibitor, similar to Prozac. I have my own theory on how this remarkable herb works.

The Sunshine Theory

Depression is a dark state of mind. People who are depressed feel blue. In fact, one particular kind of depression, seasonal affective disorder (SAD), is directly linked to lack of sunlight, and can be helped by exposure to light. Light is captured by the body as biophotons, which enhance the absorption of the sun's rays. One side effect of using St. John's wort is increased photosensitivity. This may be caused by St. John's wort's capacity to stimulate the body's production of biophotons. This also correlates with the Doctrine of Signatures as interpreted by the ancient druids, who believed that because St. John's wort blooms near the summer solstice (the longest day of the year), it is imbued with the highest intensity of sunlight. The druids considered St. John's wort to be the most sacred plant of the summer solstice; it was the physical manifestation of solar energy, frozen in time. St. John's wort can help to bring sunshine and light into your life.

Dosages	
Tea	3–5 tsp fresh or dried flowers to 1 cup water 2–3 cups per day
Tincture/Extract	2 ml 3×/day
Capsules	300mg 3×/day

St. John's wort is often standardized to 0.125–0.5% hypericin, although current research indicates that another compound, hyperforin, or perhaps a combination of both hypericin and hyperforin, may be important in its activity.

Cautions

- St. John's wort may increase photosensitivity and can cause skin rash or blisters, especially in fair skinned individuals.
- Avoid sunbathing while using St. John's wort. It may potentiate the activity of prescription MAO inhibitors.
- Be sure to tell your health care practitioner if you are using St. John's wort. It should not be taken in combination with prescription drugs.

Sea Vegetables

Sea vegetables, commonly referred to as seaweed, are full of natural minerals and vitamins. These include vitamins A, B, C, D, E, and K, as well as amino acids and essential enzymes. Seaweed is a major part of the diet of cultures around the world, including such diverse cultures as Japan and Scotland. When we consider the Doctrine of Signatures, seaweed, with its high saline content and flowing nature, reminds us of the inner fluids of the body, as well as the ebb and tide of hormones in the female cycles.

One easy way to use seaweed is to visit any Japanese restaurant. They will always have miso soup, seaweed salad, and California rolls. These all contain different kinds of seaweed. Seaweed can also be purchased in dry form in any health food store. Look for nori, arame, hijiki, and dulce. Powdered kelp, another kind of seaweed, is available as a salt substitute in convenient shake-on containers. Seaweed is particularly helpful to the endocrine system, which produces and releases hormones. Its high level of nutrients and its ability to aid in hormone balance makes it a perfect food and medicament for every aspect of the female cycle of life: menarche, menstruation, menopause, fertility, and all aspects of health, wellness, and longevity. It contains sodium alginate, which is used to offset radiation poisoning. Take extra sea vegetables whenever you are exposed to X rays.

Nutritional Powerhouse from the Sea

by Roger G. Windsor

There are hundreds of varieties of sea vegetables, all with different tastes, textures, and appearances. There are green, beige, red, brown and black ones; they come in flakes, sheets, pieces, and powders; some are twisty and noodle-shaped, or flat and chunky; all have their own distinct tastes. Sea vegetables are real power-houses of nutrition. No other foods contain the wide array of nutrients that they offer. Edible seaweeds are packed with nutrients including vitamins A , C, E, B complex, and B12, as well as calcium, potassium, iron, and trace minerals. Dried hiziki contains fourteen times the calcium of milk, and kelp contains almost every mineral and trace element required for human existence. All sea vegetables contain iodine, an essential nutrient necessary for thyroid function. The thyroid gland helps to regulate the metabolism of the cells, and the basal metabolic rate is responsible for the greatest percentage of calories expended by our bodies. Thus, a well-tuned metabolism is critical for maintaining proper weight. One of the hormones produced by the thyroid gland, thyroxine, is composed of 65 percent iodine by weight. Sea vegetables are also a rich source of non-digestible fiber which encourages the prompt elimination of toxins from the bowel and reduces the amount of time these toxins remain in our bodies. Fiber also has a positive effect on the balance of healthy flora in the intestinal tract, affecting both the composition and activity of the flora. This is important because intestinal flora not only produce beneficial nutrients needed by our bodies, they also protect against pathogens and toxins. Some sea vegetables have been studied extensively for their healing properties, such as kombu (*Laminaria*). Several studies have shown that this species has the ability to actively destroy cancer cells, as well as stimulate T-cell production in our immune systems (*Cancer Research* 44:2758-61, 1984, *Cancer Letters* 35:109-18, 1987). After World War II, numerous researchers and health care providers discovered kombu's ability to bind with radioactive isotopes in the body, thus allowing them to be safely discharged. Some varieties have potent anti-inflammatory, antiviral, antimicrobial, and antifungal properties. Sea vegetables have been used in the diets of coastal peoples around the world in Europe, Africa, and South America. They have been an especially important ingredient in Japanese and Chinese traditional medicine and cuisine. In Japan, kombu is used in fish and meat dishes and in soups, and as a vegetable with rice. The Japanese also use dulse as a cold remedy and wakame to increase hair growth and luster, and to enhance skin tone. Laver, a purplish-black sea vegetable, has been enjoyed in the British Isles for centuries, mixed with fat and rolled oats and fried into a breakfast bread in Scotland and Wales. Even now, the common food additive carrageenan, also called Irish moss, found along the west coast of Ireland and America's Atlantic coast, is used in cosmetics, medicines, and as a thickening agent for foods such as puddings, ice cream, and soups. Native Americans use one type of sea vegetable, bladderwrack, in steam baths to help alleviate the pains of rheumatism. With the growing popularity of Japanese food and restaurants, more and more people are consuming sea vegetables, even though they may not know it. The black wrapping of sushi is a sea vegetable called nori, and the dark greenish-brown pieces floating in miso soup is wakame.

Sea vegetables are easy to use. They expand to many times their original volume, so small amounts go a long way. Add them in dried form to soups, stews, and beans while they cook, but for most other recipes, always soak them in water for about 10 minutes or until soft, before cooking. Sea vegetables taste best when cooked with adequate salt, in the form of shoyu, miso, or granular sea salt. The source and quality of sea vegetables are very important. Select sea vegetables harvested from pure, pristine areas, and choose reputable brands to insure that they have not been contaminated. Sea vegetables are also classed or graded according to quality, so select the highest grade available to insure you receive the greatest benefit.

Reprinted with Permission from VitalCast.com Online Magazine, April 20, 2000

CYCLES OF LIFE

Types of Sea Vegetables

Nori is best known for its use as the outer layer of Japanese rice sushi, but pieces of toasted nori can also be used to wrap rice balls, or else nori can be cut into thin julienne strips and used to garnish noodles, grains, soups, or salads. Before use, nori sheets need to be lightly toasted over a flame (or an electric burner) for a few moments until they become slightly crisp. Ground nori makes a tasty condiment, and toasted sheets of nori make a nice, tasty snack for kids.

Wakame has a mild flavor and an attractive green color. It is used mainly in salads, miso soup and stir-fries.

Arame is a popular sea vegetable with a sweet, delicate taste. It is usually added to soups or salads, and is often sautéed with root vegetables, tofu, or soybeans.

Hijiki has a strong taste and a black, string-like appearance. It is usually cooked with tempeh or tofu, but it can also be sautéed with root vegetables, or eaten cold in salads.

Kombu is usually used either to make a broth for noodles, or else it is simmered in water and shoyu to make soup stock. Try adding a piece of kombu when you are cooking beans, and it will make them more tender and digestible. Kombu can also be cooked with tofu, tempeh, seitan, or root vegetables.

Agar flakes are often used as a setting agent for jellies or other desserts.

MISO SOUP

1 oz dried wakame
1 cup thinly sliced onions
1 qt water
½ cup miso (use less miso for a less salty taste)

Soak the wakame in water until soft. Cut into ½-inch pieces. Add onions, bring to a boil, and cook for 10 minutes. Stir up miso in a separate bowl with ¼ cup of the cooking water until pureed. Add to the soup and simmer for 5 minutes.

For more recipes see *Sea Vegetables Harvesting Guide and Cookbook* by Evelyn McConnaughey and *Seaweed: A Cook's Guide : Tempting Recipes for Seaweed and Sea Vegetables* by Lesley Ellis.

Dosage	
Seaweed	1–2 Tbs/day

Siberian Ginseng
(Eleutherococcus senticosus)

Siberian ginseng is a cousin to Chinese (Panax) ginseng. It is a shrub that grows in the forest undergrowth in Russia, Northeast China, the Japanese island of Hokkaido, and Korea. It's genus and species name means "free-berried shrub with thorns." One of its common names, "touch me not" is probably based on its thorny covering as well. Reference to the use of this plant can be traced to 2000 B.C. in China, and it was mentioned in the Chinese classic *The Divine Plowman* in 100 B.C. Its Chinese name is Ci Wu Jia. The root is the part of the plant that is used medicinally, and is harvested after it is at least two years old.

Siberian ginseng has been analyzed extensively. It has been found to contain a range of eleutherosides, flavonoids, polysaccharides, and glycosides, including beta-sitosterol. However, it does not contain ginsenocides which are found in Panax ginseng. Compared to Panax ginseng, Siberian ginseng is less expensive and less stimulating. It is often preferred for long-term use, and is especially favored for women.

Extracts of Siberian ginseng are recognized as effective drugs internationally. It is approved as a drug for humans by the Soviet Ministry of Health, and is approved in Germany as a useful tonic for weakness, fatigue, and memory problems. Siberian ginseng was given to victims of the Chernobyl nuclear accident in 1986 to ease radiation sickness. Athletes and astronauts in Russia were found to have increased stamina and reduced symptoms related to stress after using Siberian ginseng. Other studies have shown positive effects on atherosclerosis, diabetes, high blood sugar, and lung congestion. True adaptogens are herbs which are used to balance the body. In the case of Siberian ginseng, it is an adaptogen that can help raise low blood pressure or lower high blood pressure.

Mix Siberian ginseng with rosebuds for an immediate mood lift. It is useful for PMS, fatigue, headache, and mild depression associated with the menstrual cycle and menopause.

Dosages

Tea	1–2 tsp in one cup of hot water, steeped for 5 minutes
Extract/Tincture	2 ml drops 3×/day
Capsules	100–200 milligrams 2×/day

Caution

- Use with medical supervision if you have chronic hypertension.

Wild Carrot (Daucus carota)

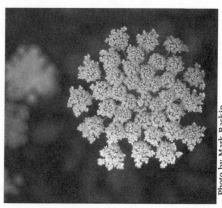

Photo by Mark Raskin

This plant is referred to by many names including "birds nest." In fact it is the main ingredient in the oriental bird's nest soup. Wild carrot grows throughout most temperate regions of the world. It can be seen along roadsides and abandoned fields. It grows over a two-year life cycle. In the first year, the leaves look just like the feathered leaves of garden variety carrots. The root is a pale yellow with a carrot-like flavor, and can be used in soups and stews. The distinctive umbrella-shaped flower appears during the second year, and gives the plant the name Queen Ann's lace. It refers to the elaborate lace collars Queen Ann was known for, and the tiny purple-red flower often found in the center of all the tiny white flowers is said to represent the loss of her head!

Small, oblong brown seeds can be gathered from the flower tops in late fall, after they dry and curl up into the "bird's nest." Folklore claims that using a strong tea made from these seeds helps to prevent pregnancy, if taken soon after sex. Scientific investigation has found that certain chemical constituents (porphyrin) in this herb cause the release of sex hormones (gonadatropins) from the pituitary gland, although no study has been done to confirm its contraceptive effect.

Dosage

Tea	1tsp dried seeds in 1 cup water or whole root cooked as soup

Wild Yam (Dioscorea spp.)

Wild yam, not related to sweet potatoes that are called yams in the United States, is a food staple throughout the many tropical and semi-tropical regions where it grows. The root of this vine-like plant is a thick starchy tuber which is unearthed and boiled to prepare it as a food. Indigenous women insist that eating a lot of wild yam helps them to space their babies. (However, they also nurse which is known to inhibit ovulation and act as a natural birth control.) Interestingly, the wild yam was for many years the sole source of plant-derived hormones produced by major pharmaceutical companies and used for the production of steroidal contraceptives, commonly known as birth control pills. The steroidal saponins (also called phytosterols), diosgenin, and botogenin were isolated from the yams by Japanese researchers in the early 1900s.

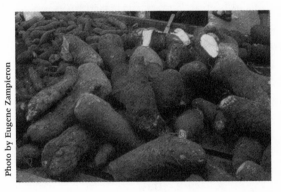

(Synthetic progesterone in an injectible form—the drug Depro-Provera—is the most widely used contraceptive on a global level.) This same plant is used for other cycles of life when increased progesterone is desired.

Photo by Eugene Zampieron

Wild Yam Creams

There is a debate in the medical community as to whether the phytosterols present in wild yam can help to increase hormone levels in the body. Many scientists explain that the prehormonal substances can only be activated in the laboratory, using enzymes and microbial transformation. Many wild yam products are available in heath food stores as cream based products that are applied transdermally (on the skin). These creams claim to help PMS, menstrual cramps, vaginal dryness, ovarian cysts, fibrocystic breasts, and other hormone related problems. They can help to restore hormonal balance to help infertility, even though yams have been used as contraceptives. They can be used during pregnancy for morning sickness and may help to avoid miscarriage. Apply to the skin directly over the uterus to help menstrual cramps and other aches and pains.

The quality and content of various brands of wild yam cream varies greatly. If the cream only contains wild yam, it is probably a good source of diosgenin, but the body cannot transform this into usable progesterone. However, many women find that these mild, less expensive creams are sufficient to help decrease symptoms. Other brands add natural progesterone and other precursor hormones such as pregnenelone, as well as cofactors that can aid in uptake and metabolism, such as vitamins B-6, B-5, A, and D-3. Some brands use an oil-based cream, while others deliver the active ingredients through a liposome system. Read product labels carefully to determine the amount of progesterone it contains per ounce. Most health care practitioners recommend creams that contain at least 400 to 500 mg of progesterone per ounce, which is higher than will be possible in a cream that contains only wild yam extract. It is best to have a test done of your progesterone levels (and other hormones including estrogen, testosterone, DHEA) before embarking on a hormonal modulating program such as the use of progesterone creams. Your health care practitioner can order hormone level tests or you can opt to do non-prescription saliva based testing (see www.salivatest.com).

Dosage

Tincture/Extract	2–3 ml 2×/day
Capsules	200–400 mg 2×/day
Cream	¼ tsp applied to breasts, arms, thighs, alternating daily. Use during days 14–28 of cycle; post-menopause, 3 weeks on, 1 off.

Caution

Wild Yam may have an additive effect with estrogenic drugs. Consult your health care practitioner.

Yan Hou Su (Corydalis yanhusuo, C. bulbosa, C. ambigua)

Pain is a universal phenomenon. Societies around the globe have experimented with many plants to discover which ones are most useful for pain relief. In traditional Chinese medicine, the top herb for pain is *Cordydalis*.

Corydalis is a shade loving perennial with golden colored tubers—rootlike structures which contains the medicinal components. It is a member of the poppy family, along with opium, and is a source of strong pain killing compounds. However, *Corydalis* does not contain morphine and it is nonaddictive. The roots contain other powerful alkaloids such as corydaline and corybulbine.

It is commonly used for menstrual cramps, postpartum pain, stomach ache, arthritis, fibromyalgia or pain in the lower back, head, neck, or shoulders. It also helps with the mental and emotional anxiety, duress, and insomnia which can accompany pain. Western research has validated the excellent pain relieving ability of *Corydalis*. It is 40 percent as effective as morphine and one tenth as strong as opium. It has earned the nickname "Chinese herbal pain killer" or "Chinese aspirin" even though it does not work via the same biochemical mechanism as aspirin, nor does it destroy the stomach like aspirin. In fact, it actually *protects* the gastrointestinal tract from damage.

It is often mixed with herbs like cinnamon, licorice root, angelica, lovage, and peony. It is available as a Chinese patent medicine formula Yan Hu Suo Zhi Tong Pain in Chinese apothecaries and is part of the formula *BotanoDyne* (see www.naturesanswer.com).

Dosage	
Dried root	minimum of 5 grams/day

Cautions

- Do not use in pregnancy.
- Do not drive or operate heavy machinery until you have a sense of how *Corydalis* affects you.

Part III

Energy

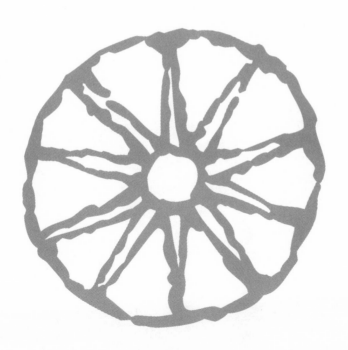

CHAPTER TEN

Circadian Rhythms

with contributions by Glen Rein, Ph.D.

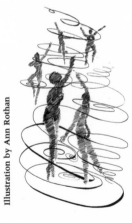

Illustration by Ann Rothan

Circadian rhythms are natural cycles within the body that are experienced by all living things. They are like spirals within spirals, interacting with each other and the individual in endless cycles. Circadian rhythms which repeat over a twenty-four-hour cycle are commonly studied. However, there are also cycles which last only a few hours, such as the sleep cycle, and others which last for days, such as the menstrual cycle (twenty-eight days in most women). Other cycles occur at different times of the year, during different seasons. In addition to the reproductive system, many other systems in the body undergo this cyclic behavior including the nervous, immune, endocrine, and cardiovascular systems. Many body functions exhibit cycles: eating, sleeping, body temperature, blood pressure, alertness, and mood.

CYCLES OF LIFE

FACTORS THAT INFLUENCE CIRCADIAN RHYTHMS

Internal Factors

Cell Structures and Chemicals. In all of nature, the microcosm is reflected by the macrocosm. If isolated cells are examined, we find that a pattern of cyclic behavior can be measured in both specific cell structures and their chemicals makeup. One hormone, melatonin, is a good example of this. Melatonin normally exists in specialized cells in the pineal gland. When pineal cells are removed from the body and kept under constant conditions, without the normal external cycle of light and dark, the amount of melatonin that is produced has a free-running cycle that is different than the one the cells follow while they are in the pineal gland. This means that cells have an intrinsic cycle of their own. Scientists believe that this intrinsic cyclic behavior of pineal cells in the brain, as well as other specialized cells throughout the body, acts like a time keeper or pacemaker. We therefore have many internal clocks ticking away at different rates, thereby accounting for the different cycles (those less than twenty-four hours and those greater than twenty-four hours) that are occurring simultaneously in our bodies.

External Factors

> The earth's rhythms hold us in an inescapable
> embrace; our connection to them is fundamental.
> —Sidney MacDonald Baker, M.D.,
> *The Circadian Prescription*

Daylight Cycles and Entrainment

The specialized cells containing the pacemaking clocks generate natural intrinsic rhythms that are affected by the environment. The daylight cycle is one of the strongest external rhythms which profoundly effects our internal cycles. External rhythms can override our intrinsic cycles. The experiments discussed above done with isolated pineal cells show that the intrinsic rhythm of the melatonin in these cells is not twenty-four hours. Yet, since the light/dark twenty-four-hour cycle is so strong, the intrinsic melatonin cycle *becomes* a twenty-four-hour cycle. This phenomenon, where the stronger cycle takes over the weaker cycle, is called entrainment, whereby external and internal cycles are synchronized. An interesting example of entrainment can be seen when groups of women, such as family members or coworkers, begin to have monthly cycles at the same time or within a few days of each other. Although modern western scientists have only recently discovered the entrainment phenomena, it has been well-known in other cultures for hundreds of years. Chinese medicine and astrology are two examples of systems that have long recognized the importance of external forces on our internal cycles.

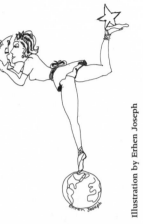

Illustration by Erhen Joseph

Other Natural Factors

Many natural environmental factors can influence our cycles. Geomagnetic fields, barometric pressure, gravity, moon cycles, sunspot activity, and other forces cause changes in our structure and chemistry which can change internal rhythms.

Human Influenced Factors

During the last century we have added the stress of manmade electromagnetic energy from a multitude of sources. These include microwave ovens, cell phones, computers, powerlines, and artificial lighting. All of these factors can have an effect on our health. If either the internal or the external cycles are thrown off in some way we may become ill. Strong cycles are associated with health whereas weak and altered cycles are associated with disease. The aging process, flying in airplanes, and working on changing shifts are examples of conditions that adversely effect circadian rhythms.

Power line influence has been studied by scientists. They observed that people who live near power lines often have similar symptoms to people with altered melatonin rhythms. After further study it was determined that weak EM (electromagnetic) fields can effect cardiovascular, neurotransmitter, and melatonin cycles.

Artificial lighting disrupts the natural light/dark cycle of nature, but artificial light can also be used to reset our clocks when they become desynchronized. Seasonal affective disorder (SAD), also called winter depression, is a condition caused by abnormal rhythms of melatonin due to lack of exposure to daylight during winter months. Symptoms include mood disturbances, insomnia, headaches, fatigue, digestive problems, and increased susceptibility to colds and flus. Scientists have discovered that people with SAD, when exposed to bright white light for two to three hours in the early morning, show a resynchronization of their melatonin cycles and a marked alleviation of their emotional and physical symptoms. Thus, external lighting sources, when applied at the right time can reestablish normal, healthy cycles. Depending on how light is used, it can either synchronize or desynchronize melatonin circadian rhythm.

MEASURING CIRCADIAN RHYTHMS

Dr. Gunther Hildebrandt performed an experiment where he compared overall fitness to rhythmic harmony based on measuring respiration and pulse rate.[22] He found that if the pulse rate divided by the respiration rate generated a whole number, the person was in better fitness condition than people whose rates generated an uneven number.

Circadian Rhythms

You may want to try this exercise before and after using specific stress-reduction techniques such as deep breathing, yoga, meditation, or even a soothing aromatherapy bath. These practices can help bring your rhythms into balance. Don't allow your numbers, if not always whole, to add to your stress level! Simply accept it as an indicator on your path to deeper self understanding.

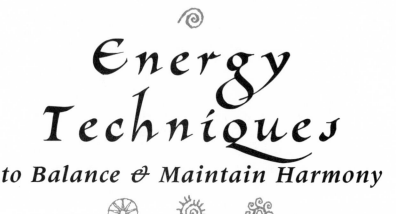

CHAPTER ELEVEN

Energy Techniques

to Balance & Maintain Harmony

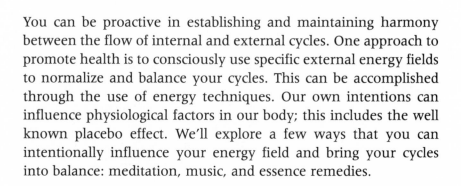

You can be proactive in establishing and maintaining harmony between the flow of internal and external cycles. One approach to promote health is to consciously use specific external energy fields to normalize and balance your cycles. This can be accomplished through the use of energy techniques. Our own intentions can influence physiological factors in our body; this includes the well known placebo effect. We'll explore a few ways that you can intentionally influence your energy field and bring your cycles into balance: meditation, music, and essence remedies.

THE POWER OF INTENTION

"Intentionality" research is a new area of science that investigates how human intention can be directed to influence specific biological processes. An exciting study by Dr. Glen Rein, Ph.D.,[23] clearly demonstrates that focusing your conscious mind can either cause DNA strands to wind or unwind. Dr. Rein concluded that when test subjects were able to synchronize their heart and mind, determined by measuring EKG and EEG patterns, they could successfully wrap or unwrap DNA strands at will! Further research in this area will lead to our understanding more about the unlimited healing capacity we all have available to us!

THE PLACEBO EFFECT

The power of the mind is acknowledged in conventional medicine, where it is called the placebo effect. A placebo is an inactive substance, such as a sugar pill, which is often used alongside an active substance, such as a drug, to see how much effect the drug actually has. The use of the double blind placebo control trial has been the gold standard for proving the efficacy of certain pharmaceutical agents. The well documented placebo effect collaborates the power of the mind in healing. The placebo effect is thought to work through three mechanisms:

- conditioning
- endorphin release
- expectation

For instance, if people are given sugar water and are told it is an emetic they will often vomit. The placebo response rate can be quite high—up to 80 percent in some experiments![24] Scientists involved in testing the efficacy of drugs often find the placebo effect to be an annoyance that interferes with research. But perhaps we should honor and extol this effect and use it to its maximum potential in our own self healing.

MEDITATION

Scientific studies have confirmed that meditation reduces stress and has beneficial effects on the body.[25] Could it be that these beneficial effects are brought about by the re-synchronization of our rhythms?

Energy Techniques

INSTANT MEDITATION

Find a quiet place. Loosen the clothing around your waist. Close your eyes. Breath in deeply and allow your lower abdomen to expand. Hold the breath for two seconds, then exhale slowly. Continue this breathing pattern for five minutes. Allow your mind to focus on your breath. If other thoughts intrude, just gently allow them to pass. Aromatherapy is a wonderful adjunct to meditation. Use any essential oil or incense that you find pleasing. Sandalwood, patchouli, rose, and lavender are some suggestions. Sprinkle a few drops on a tissue and inhale the scent each time you meditate. It can help to train your mind to return quickly to the peaceful healing pattern of meditation. For instance, simply inhaling the aroma of the essential oil you use for meditation can return you to a peaceful state of mind during other times of the day.

MUSIC
(with contributions by Steven Angel, D.C.)

We all know from experience that music has the ability to affect both emotions and moods, sometimes with exceptionally powerful results. Various forms of music have very predictable effects on human behavior. Marching music creates entrainment—uniting soldiers marching into war or stirring the emotions of spectators during sports events. Certain types of music are appropriate for specific purposes. Research continues to confirm the healing power of music. Patients with Parkinson's disease, for example, show improvements in physical, behavioral, and emotional symptoms with music therapy.[26]

Studies have shown that music of a meditative nature can lower blood pressure as well as reduce the level of stress hormones. Dr. Mockel and several coworkers at the Free University of Berlin experimented with three types of music to determine their effects on hormonal levels.[27] The three kinds of music used for the study were:

- Ravi Shankar's meditative music—without strong rhythmic characteristics
- Johann Strauss—a waltz with a strong rhythm
- W. H. Henze—another classical piece

The outcome was that Ravi Shanker's music reduced cortisol and noradrenaline secretions significantly.

I did a study on 100 patients comparing the effects of Steven Halpern's *Crystal Suite* with the sound of a leaf blower. The outcome showed that listening to Steven Halpern's music increased the activity of white blood cells (part of the immune system), while the sound of the leaf blower inhibited white blood cell activity. (Steven's music is extremely relaxing and healing; see www.stevenhalpern.com.)

Some types of music, especially those which are more meditative in nature, can help you reduce stress hormones, especially cortisol and noradrenaline, and benefit your immune system function. More research is needed in this field, but feel free to experiment with different kinds of music. See which ones cheer you up, relax you, or get you going. Then consciously use music as a healing and balancing tool.

ESSENCE REMEDIES

Essence remedies work by balancing your emotions. The term *psychoneuroimmunology*, coined by Dr. Candace Pert, describes the intricate network within our bodies where specific chemicals called neurotransmitters are released in response to every thought and action we experience. This influences our entire physiology in a profound manner. The function of the immune system, cellular use of oxygen, and the release of specific hormones are a few examples of how these powerful forces effect our bodies.

Essence remedies are extremely subtle and gentle, yet incredibly powerful in their effect. I often recommend that people start with essence remedies as they begin their path of experimentation with natural healing substances, since they can be safely used by anyone at any age regardless of other medications and physical conditions. Essence remedies are prepared by capturing the essence of naturally occurring products and processes in water and preserving the fluid with a small amount of alcohol.

It is not within the scope of this book to outline exactly which of the essence remedies to use for different emotional and physical conditions. My intent here is to bring the knowledge of this simple self-care system to your awareness, so that you can pursue it if you feel so inspired. Essence remedies are the domain of *any* woman!

Bach Remedies

Dr. Edmond Bach, a physician practicing in the early 1900s, believed that every illness had an emotional component as a root cause. For true healing to occur, this emotional component needed to be addressed and balanced. He came to this conclusion long before the term psychoneuroimmunology was coined. He also noted that plants and flowers were intimately connected to our emotional states. Flowers have always been used to honor emotional occasions such as weddings and funerals. Trees can bring a sense of stability and grounding. He began to experiment with making remedies from various plants and flowers and trying them on himself and others—a system called *proving*. He noticed that specific plants had a pattern of association with specific emotions. He developed his original twelve essence remedies described in his book *The Twelve Healers*. The Bach flower remedy line now consists of thirty-six remedies plus the well known Rescue Remedy (a combination product), an excellent adjunct to anyone's natural medicine chest!

Bach remedies are available in most health food stores. Here is an example of how remedies can be used: Combine 7 drops of the desired remedy in a little water—for adults or children. Sip the mixture several times throughout the day. You might want to try the following:

- *for fear,* aspen, mimulus,
- *for depression,* gentian, rock rose
- *for low self-esteem,* oak, vine, vervain
- *for loneliness,* gorse, water violet

After you have tried the commercially prepared Bach remedies, you may want to prepare your own essence remedies. The best kind of water to use is natural spring water. However, there is an ironic side to bottled spring water. In order to be labeled as spring water it must be infused with chlorine to kill bacteria, then the chlorine is filtered out. One brand of water that is not subject to this process is Trinity Springs Water (see www.trinitysprings.com). This water is taken from a source over two miles deep in rural Idaho. It percolates through quartz crystal caverns and is truly living water. The bottle states that it is a dietary supplement. Since it does not claim to be spring water, it avoids the mandatory adding of chlorine. This brand of water is wonderful to use to make your own essence remedies. Good filtered water will also work.

TRADITIONAL FLOWER ESSENCE PREPARATION

To prepare your remedy, go outside and find a beautiful flower that inspires you. Cut the flower and let it fall into a glass vessel filled with water. Allow the sunlight to infuse into the water for several hours. Remove the plant material with a wooden spoon. Add 1 teaspoon brandy per pint of water to preserve the remedy. Store in a dark amber bottle in a cool dry place.

Himalayan Remedies

There are many other essence remedies besides Bach remedies. Two physicians from India, Drs. Atul and Rupa Shah, have created the Himalayan remedies (see www.aumhimalaya.com). These remedies are prepared from exotic flowers from the Himalayan mountains which are infused into sacred filtered water from the Ganges River. Drs. Shah are western trained medical physicians who have dedicated their lives to the study of the effect of subtle energy on human health and wellness. Their remedies deal with deeper levels of psychological and spiritual imbalances, such as dealing with rejection and criticism or deep spiritual longing.

Besides remedies made from flowers, they have gemstone essence remedies and many subtle energy devices that can help deal with electromagnetic pollution and other ravages of modern life. They have created an interesting method of preparing remedies that you may want to try.

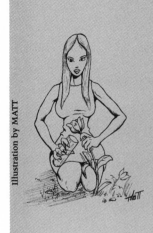

Illustration by MATT

LIVE FLOWER REMEDY PREPARATION:

After you identify your special flower, don't cut it off the plant. Instead, bend the flower gently into a tall glass container. Try not to crush or damage it in any way. Then pour spring water over the flower until it is completely immersed. Allow sunlight to infuse the water for 5 to 10 minutes, or until you feel the essence is captured. Then gently remove the flower from the glass of water without damaging it. You now have your "mother essence." Add brandy to preserve. Store in a dark amber bottle in a cool dry place.

Perelandra Remedies

Machaelle Small Wright, author of *Co-Creative Science, Behaving as if the God in All Life Mattered* (and other books), has created the Perelandra remedies named after her magical garden in Virginia (see www.perelandra-ltd.com). Her remedies address very deep issues. Examples are:

- Cauliflower—Stabilizes and balances the child during the birth process.
- Comfrey—Repairs higher vibrational soul damage that has occurred in the present or a past lifetime.
- Zinnia—Reconnects one to the child within. Restores playfulness, laughter, joy, and a sense of healthy priorities.

Gemstone Remedies

Essence remedies can be made from many other sources besides flowers. Gemstone elixirs are available commercially or can be prepared at home. Gemstone elixirs often address spiritual growth. Examples include:

- Amethyst—Increased spiritual awareness.
- Clear Quartz—Focused intention and clarity of purpose.
- Turquoise—Connection to ancient ancestors.
- Malachite—Slowing down and paying attention.

PREPARING A GEMSTONE REMEDY

Allow a gemstone of your choice to soak in a glass container filled with water in the sunlight for a few hours. Remove the gemstone from the water with a wooden spoon.

Imponderables

Imponderables are remedies that are made by capturing the essence of natural phenomena, such as an inspiring thunderstorm or the summer solstice. You can also use this method to save the essence of a special occasion, such as a wedding or birthday. To make your own, set a jar of water in a location in the midst of the event, such as out in the thunderstorm or on the altar during a wedding ceremony. Then hold your hands around the jar and project your intention to preserve the energy of the event into the water. Maintain your attention to this for five minutes. Then allow the jar to stay put for several hours.

PRESERVING YOUR REMEDY

Whether you use the Bach, Himalayan, Gemstone, or Imponderable methods, when your remedy is complete add some unflavored brandy to your water solution. Use about 1 tablespoon of brandy to 4 ounces of remedy.

USING HOMEMADE REMEDIES

When you use a commercially prepared remedy, it will come with an instruction manual that will guide you as to the use for each individual remedy. If you are new to this it is useful to use these prepared remedies along with the instructions. When preparing your own remedies you need to access your own innate intelligence. This process of opening and allowing in an influx of subtle information is a female process, whether performed by a man or a woman. At times the answer seems obvious—a thunderstorm remedy can help a person through a tumultuous period. When I asked a friend what her newly made gladiolus remedy was for, she answered, "Well, of course, it makes one feel glad!" There is no wrong use for a self-made remedy.

When you are ready to work with your new remedy, take a moment to center, breathing in deeply and slowly seven times. Tell your mind that your intention is to have an insight about how this remedy might best be used. Simply hold the bottle containing the remedy, and place a small amount of the water solution under your tongue and on the skin of your wrists. Have a clean, blank piece of paper ready or a blank computer screen. Breath in deeply again while you simply allow thoughtforms or feelings to enter your consciousness. Then record whatever comes to mind. Do not analyze, censor, or try to figure out any of the incoming information. Just record it. It may come in as one word, a sentence, or a full paragraph or more. Don't sit for too long, 10 to 15 minutes is sufficient. Put what you wrote away. Review it later or even in a few days. If it feels correct, it is!

Notes

1. Corsello, Serafina. *The Ageless Women.* City: Publisher, Date. 154.
2. Barnes, S.; Sfakianos, J.; Coward, L.; Kirk, M. "Soy isoflavonoids and cancer prevention. Underlying biochemical and pharmacological issues." *Adv Exp Med Biol.* 1996; 401: 87–100.
3. Native American Dance—National Museum of the American Indian. Smithsonian Institute, Washington, DC, 1993.
4. Peters, P. H., et.al., "Age at Menarche and Breast Cancer Risk in Nulliparous Women" *Breast Cancer Research and Treatment.* 1995; 33(1): 55–61
5. Hochschild, Arlie, and Ann MacHung. *The Second Shift.* City: Publisher, Date.
6. Abraham, G., M.D. "Nutritional Factors in the etiology of the premenstrual tension syndromes." *Journal of Reproductive Medicine.* 1983; 28: 452.
7. Seibel, M. *Infertility, A Comprehensive Text,* East Norwalk, Conn.: Appleton & Lange, 1990, 7–9.
8. Gibson R. A., Neumann M. A., Makrides M. "Effect of dietary docosahexaenoic acid on brain composition and neural function in term infants." *Lipids,* 1996; 31: 177S–181S.
9. Garry, D., Figueroa, R., et al. "Use of Castor Oil in Pregnancies at Term," *Alternative Therapies in Health and Medicine,* Jan 2000; 6: 1.
10. Hawton, K., Gath, D., Day, A. "Sexual function in a community sample of middle-aged women with partners: effects of age, marital, socioeconomic, psychiatric, gynecological, and menopausal factors." *Arch Sex Behav.* Aug 1994; 23(4): 375–395.
11. Beard, M. K. "Atrophic vaginitis. Can it be prevented?" *Post Graduate Medicine,* May 1992; 91: 257.
12. DeAngelis, Lissa, and Molly Simple. *Recipes for Change, Gourmet Wholefood Cooking for Health and Vitality.* City: Publisher, Date.

13. Zampieron, E., Kamhi, E. *The Natural Medicine Chest*. New York: M. Evans, 1999, 107.
14. Duker, E. M., et. al. "Effects of extracts from Cimicifuga racemosa on gonadotropin release in menopausal women and ovariectomized rats." *Planta Medica*, 1991; 57: 420–424.
15. Garry, D., Figueroa, R, et al. "Use of Castor Oil in Pregnancies at Term," *Alternative Therapies in Health and Medicine*, Jan 2000; 6: 1.
16. Diehm, C., et al. "Comparison of leg compression stockings and oral horse chestnut extract therapy in patients with CVI." *The Lancet*, 1996; 347: 292. Pittler, M. H., et al. "Horse chestnut seed extract for chronic venous insufficiency." *Arch Dermatol*, 1998; 134.
17. Pittler, M. H., Ernst, E. "Efficacy of kava extract for treating anxiety: systematic review and meta-analysis," *J Clin Psychopharmacol*. Feb. 2000; 20(1): 84–89.
18. Kamhi, E., Zampieron, E. "Licorice Root for Inflammation," *Inter Jour of Integrative Medicine*, May 2000; 2: 30–32.
19. Ibid.
20. Miller, D. A. *Forage Crops*. New York: McGraw Hill, 1984.
21. Volz, H. P., Laux, P. "Potential treatment for sub-threshold and mild depression: a comparison of St. John's wort extracts and fluoxetine." *Comparative Psychiatry*. Mar/Apr 2000;41(2 Suppl 1):133–137.
22. Hildebrandt, Gunther, *Basis of an Individual Physiology: a new image of man in medicine*. City: Publisher, Date.
23. Rein, G. "Effect of Conscious Intention on Human DNA." International Forum on New Science, Denver, Colo., Oct 1996.
24. Harrington, A., ed. *The Placebo Effect; an Interdisciplinary Exploration*. Cambridge, Masss: Harvard University Press, 1997, 12–36.
25. Harmon, R. L.; Myers, M. A. "Prayer and meditation as medical therapies." *Phys Med Rehabil Clin N Am*. Aug 1999; 10(3): 651–662.
26. Pacchetti, C., Mancini, F., et al. "Active music therapy in Parkinson's disease: an integrative method for motor and emotional rehabilitation," *Psychosomatic Med*. 2000; 62: 386–393.
27. Mokel, M., Rocker, L., et al. "Immediate physiological responses of healthy volunteers to different types of music:cardiovascular, hormonal and mental changes," *Eur J Appl Physiol*, 1994; 68: 451–459.

Symptom Cross Reference

Aches and pains—black cohosh, blue cohosh, burdock, dong guai, ho shu wu, kava kava, licorice root, nettle, sea vegetables

Acne—burdock, damiana, dandelion, green foods, ho shu wu, milk thistle, oats, red clover

Alopecia (hair loss)—castor oil, green foods, ho shu wu, oats

Anemia—dandelion, dong guai, ho shu wu, green foods, milk thistle, motherwort, nettle, red clover, sea vegetables

Anxiety—black cohosh, chamomile, damiana, kava kava, motherwort, St. John's wort

Aphrodisiac—damiana, oats, kava kava, sea vegetables

Asthma—blue cohosh, dong guai, motherwort

Avoid when pregnant—black cohosh (early), blue cohosh, chaste berry, dong guai, licorice root, motherwort, rue, wild yam, *and any herb, unless a knowledgeable health care practitioner is consulted*

Birth—black cohosh, blue cohosh, burdock, castor oil, dong quai, kava kava, motherwort, nettle, red raspberry, Jamaican dogwood

CYCLES OF LIFE

Blood sugar—fenugreek, Siberian ginseng

Breast cysts—burdock, castor oil, dandelion, green foods, milk thistle, red clover, sea vegetables, wild yam

Ceremony—black cohosh, damiana, red clover, rue, rosebud

Contraceptive—burning bush, castor oil, rue, wild carrot, wild yam

Depression—damiana, green foods, kava kava, oats, rosebud, sea vegetables, Siberian ginseng, St. John's wort

Diuretic—burdock, dandelion, false unicorn root, motherwort, nettle

Endometriosis—burdock, chaste berry, dandelion, milk thistle, nettle, red clover, sea vegetables, wild yam

Epilepsy—blue cohosh, motherwort

Fatigue—deer antler, ho shu wu, green foods, milk thistle, nettle, oats, sea vegetables, Siberian ginseng, wild yam

Headache—damiana, dong quai, kava kava, nettle, rosebuds, Siberian ginseng, St. John's wort, wild yams, Jamaican dogwood

Heart—dong quai, motherwort, sea vegetables

High blood pressure—blue cohosh, dong quai, motherwort

Hot flashes—black cohosh, burdock, dandelion, dong quai, motherwort, red clover, sea vegetables, wild yams

Infertility—black cohosh, chaste berry, damiana, dong quai, false unicorn root, green beans, green foods, ho shu wu, motherwort, red raspberry, sea vegetables, wild yams

Insomnia—black cohosh, chamomile, kava kava, motherwort, sea vegetables

Irritability—black cohosh, burdock, chamomile, damiana, dong quai, kava kava, motherwort, sea vegetables, St. John's wort

Symptom Cross Reference

Kidney—burdock, damiana, dandelion, false unicorn root, ho shu wu, motherwort, nettle

Labor pain—blue cohosh, kava kava, motherwort, Jamaican dogwood

Laxative—cascara sagrada, castor oil, damiana, ho shu wu

Liver—burdock, dandelion, false unicorn root, ho shu wu, licorice root, milk thistle

Lymphatic system—burdock, castor oil, dandelion, green foods, ho shu wu, nettle, red clover, sea vegetables, oats

Menopause—black cohosh, chaste berry, dong quai, ho shu wu, licorice root, milk thistle, motherwort, nettle, red clover, sea vegetables, Siberian ginseng, wild yam

Menstrual cramps—black cohosh, chamomile, corydalis yan hoo su, dong quai, kava kava, motherwort, red raspberry, rosebuds, sea vegetables, St. John's wort, wild yam, Jamaican dogwood

Menstrual flow balance—black cohosh, blue cohosh, burdock, burning bush as floralbus (homeopathic), chaste berry, damiana, dong quai, licorice root, motherwort, nettle, red clover, red raspberry, sea vegetables, Siberian ginseng, wild yam

Nausea/morning sickness—ginger, red raspberry, wild yam

Nursing—black cohosh, chaste berry, fennel seeds, fenugreek, green foods, milk thistle, nettle, oats, red raspberry

Osteoporosis—black cohosh, green foods, ho shu wu, sea vegetables

Ovarian cysts—burdock, castor oil, dandelion, green foods, milk thistle, red clover, sea vegetables, wild yam

PMS—chaste berry, dandelion, dong quai, kava kava, licorice root, milk thistle, motherwort, red clover, sea vegetables, Siberian ginseng, wild yam

Postpartum pain—black cohosh, corydalis, kava kava, motherwort, red raspberry, sea vegetables, St. John's wort, wild yam, yan hoo su, Jamaican dogwood

Pregnancy—green foods, nettle, oats, red raspberry, sea vegetables

Radiation—sea vegetables, Siberian ginseng

Sedative—black cohosh, chamomile, dong quai, Jamaican dogwood, kava kava, motherwort, red clover, St. John's wort

Skin—burdock, castor oil, dandelion, green foods, milk thistle, nettle, oats, red clover, sea vegetables

Stomach—chamomile, licorice (DGL), milk thistle, motherwort (bitter)

Tonic—burdock, green foods, ho shu wu, nettle, oats, red raspberry, sea vegetables, Siberian ginseng,

Urinary tract—burdock, burning bush as floralbus (homeopathic), damiana, dandelion, false unicorn root, motherwort, nettle

Vaginal dryness—black cohosh, castor oil, dong quai, sea vegetables, wild yam

Varicose veins—gotu kola, horse chestnut, red raspberry

Yeast infections—tea tree oil, acidophilus

Resources

ORGANIZATIONS

American Association of Naturopathic Physicians
PO Box 20386
Seattle, WA 98012
206-323-7610
To find a licensed doctor of naturopathic medicine.

American Herbalist's Guild
1931 Gaddis Road
Canton, Georgia 30115
770-751-6021
fax: 770-751-7472
email: ahgoffice@earthlink.net
web : www.healthy.net/herbalists
A professional organization of clinical and traditional herbalists; grants the title AHG; recognized as the only national professional herbalist certification in the U.S.

American Holistic Nurse's Association
PO Box 2130
Flagstaff, Arizona 86003-2130
800-278-AHNA
web: www.ahna.org
For information on becoming or finding a holistic nurse.

Couple to Couple League
PO Box 111184
Cincinnati, OH 45211
513-471-2000
web: www.ccli.org
For information on the sympto-thermal method of birth control.

TESTS

Fern Test Equipment
PFT 1-2-3
Chain Reactions, Inc.
11230 Gold Express Drive, Building 310, #272
Gold River, CA 95672
916-944-4009

Ovu-Tech
911 N.W. 30th Ave.
Ocala, FL 34475
888-337-6464

Saliva Test for Hormones
Aeron LifeCycles
1933 Davis Street, Suite 310
San Leandro, CA 94577
800-631-7900

Sabre Sciences, EndoScreen Labs
910 Hampshire Road, Suite A
Westlake Village, CA 91361
888-490-7300

ECOTOURISM

EcoTours for Cures, The Education Vacation
PO Box 525
Oyster Bay, NY 11771
800-829-0918
web: www.naturalnurse.com

Resources

Tour Leaders: Eugene R. Zampieron, N.D., AHG, Ethnobotanist; Ellen Kamhi, Ph.D., R.N.—The Natural Nurse; Jamba, Maroon Bush Doctor; Kibret Neguse, musician.

Explore the rainforests; travel with shaman and indigenous healers and discover their medicines; experience traditional music, foods, and culture; EcoTours for Cures leads travelers on ecotravel adventures to pristine, indigenous areas of Jamaica, Costa Rica, and Belize.

Understanding Chinese Medicine: A Personalized Tour of Chinatown, New York City
> PO Box 525
> Oyster Bay, NY 11771
> 800-829-0918

Ongoing one day seminars in New York City's Chinatown with a focus on Chinese herbology.

MAGAZINES

Alternative Medicine
> 21½ Main Street
> Tiburon , CA 94920
> 800-333-HEAL
> web: www.alternativemedicine.com

The voice of alternative medicine. In-depth articles and information.

Healthy and Natural Journal
> 100 Wallace Ave
> Suite 100
> Sarasota, Fl 34237
> 888-349-4959
> web: www.healthyandnatural.com

The Natural Medicine Chest column by Eugene Zampieron and Ellen Kamhi. Articles, information, and resources for all aspects of natural living.

Herbal Gram Magazine
> PO Box 201660
> Austin, Texas 78720
> (512) 331-8868

Published by the American Botanical Council and the Herb Research Foundation. Up-to-date scientific, medical, and political information about herbal medicine.

New Living
>   1212 Route 25A, Suite 1B
>   Stony Brook, NY 11790
>   1-800-639-5484
>   email: charvey@newliving.com
>   web: www.newliving.com

Excellent monthly publication on health and fitness.

HERB SOURCES

Frontier Herbs
>   Norway, IA 52318
>   800-669-3275

Growers and providers of fresh and dried organic bulk herbs.

Horizon Herbs
>   PO Box 69
>   Williams, OR 97544
>   541-846-6704
>   email: herbseed@chatlink.com

Source of seeds for medicinal plants.

Nature's Answer
>   320 Oser Ave.
>   Hauppauge, NY 11788
>   800-439-2324
>   www.naturesanswer.com

Manufacturers of holistically balanced herbal products, including a special line of arthritis herbal products with many exotic botanicals, co-designed by the author, *The ArthroNutrition Program.*

Original Swiss Aromatics
>   PO Box 6842
>   San Rafael, CA 94903
>   415-479-9120
>   fax: 415-479-0614

High quality essential oils.

Resources

OTHER INFORMATION AVAILABLE
FROM THE AUTHOR

Natural Alternatives Health, Education and Multimedia Services
PO Box 525
Oyster Bay, NY 11771
800-829-0918
email: naturalalt@juno.com
web: www.naturalnurse.com

Natural Alternative's Herbal Workshops
with Ellen Kamhi, *The Natural Nurse,* and Eugene Zampieron, N.D.
800-829-0918
web: www.naturalnurse.com
Call for updated schedule

Environmental Detoxification Consultants & Products
PO Box 525
Oyster Bay, NY 11771
203-263-2970
email: ezkpz@juno.com
Water filtration, air purification, and environmental screening tests for toxic exposure and allergies; consultation and detoxification programs developed.

MEDIA SCHEDULE

Radio

WUSB 90.1 FM Fri.	6–7 P.M.	(or on www.wusb.org)
WPKN 89.5 FM Alt. Sun.	8–9 A.M.	(CT and Long Island, NY)
WHPC 90.3 FM Tues.	6:30–7 P.M.	(Long Island, NY)

Television

Channel 12 News, Thursdays (Long Island, NY)
Ask The Family Doctor, America's Health Network (check local listings www.ahn.com)

ESSENCE REMEDIES

Himalayan Remedies

Aum Himalaya Sanjeevini Essences
15 Em Jai Bharat Society, 3rd Road, Khar West
Mumbai (Bombay)-400 052 INDIA
648 68 19/604 75 29
fax: (00-91-22) 605 09 75
email: rupaatul@bom3.vsnl.net.in
web: www.aumhimalaya.com

Perelandra

PO Box 3603
Warrenton, VA 20188
U.S. & Canada Order Line: 1-800-960-8806
Overseas or Mexico Order Line: 1-540-937-2153
fax: 1-540-937-3360
email: email@perelandra-ltd.com
web: http://www.perelandra-ltd.com

Bibliography

Albo, Shana. *Infertility Solutions: Natural Approaches*. New York, NY: Avery Publishers, 2000.

Baker, Sidney. *The Circadian Prescription*. New York, NY: Penquin Putnum Inc., 2000.

Bentky, Virginia Williams. *Let Herbs Do It*. Boston: Houghton Mifflin, 1973.

Berger, Judith. *Herbal Rituals*. New York: St. Martin's Press, 1998.

Bianchini, Corbetta, Pistola. *Health Plants of the World*. New York: Newsweek Books, 1970.

Blumenthal, Mark. *The Complete German Commission E. Monographs: Therapeutic Guide to Herbal Medicines*. Boston, MA: American Botanical Council, 1998

Bremness, Lesley. *Herbs*. New York: Dorling Kindersley, 1994.

Brill, "Wildman" Steve. *Identifying & Harvesting Edible and Medicinal Plants in Wild and not so Wild Places*. New York: Hearst Books, 1994.

Burn, Barbara. *North American Wildflowers*. New York: Bonanza Books, 1984.

Corsello, Searfina. *The Ageless Women*. New York, NY: Corsello Communications, Inc., 1999.

Chevallier, Andrew. *The Encyclopedia of Medicinal Plants*. New York: Dorling Kindersley, 1996.

Christopher, John. *School of Natural Healing*. Provo, Utah: Christopher Publishing, 1976.

Clark, Linda. *Handbook of Natural Remedies for Common Ailments*. New York: Simon & Shuster, 1976.

Crellin, John, and Jane Philpott. *A Reference Guide to Medicinal Plants.* Durham, N.C.:Duke University Press, 1990.

Culpepper, Nicholas. *Culpepper's Herbal Remedies.* Wilshire, CA: Wilshire Book Company, 1971.

D'Amelio, Sr. *Botanicals, A Phytogesic Desk Reference.* Boca Raton, FL: CRC Press, 1999

DeAngelis, Lissa and Molly Siple. *Recipes for Change: Gourmet Whole Foods Cooking for Health and Vitality at Menopause.* New York, NY: Penguin Books, 1996.

Demargaux, D.N., *Phytotherapy.* Surrey, England: Herbal Health Publishers, 1989

Densmore, F. *How Indians Use Wild Plants for Food, Medicine and Crafts.* New York: Dover Publications, 1984.

Dunas, Felice. *Passion Play.* New York, NY: Riverhead Books, 1997.

Elliot, Doug. *Wild Roots.* Rochester, Vt: Healing Arts Press, 1995.

Flynn, Rebecca and Mark Roest. *Your Guide To Standardized Herbal Products.* Prescott, AZ: One World Press, 1995.

Foster, Steven. *Herbs For Your Health.* Loveland, CO: Interweave Press, 1996.

Grellin, John and Jane Phillpott. *A Reference Guide to Medicinal Plants.* Durham, NC: Duke University Press, 1990.

Goldberg, Burton. *Women's Health Series I and II.* Tiburon, CA: Alternativemedicine.com Books, 1998

Goldstein, Steven. *The Estrogen Alternative.* New York, NY: Berkeley Publishing Book, 1998.

Griggs, Barbara, *Green Pharmacy.* Rochester, N.Y.: Healing Arts Press, 1996.

_____.*The Green Witch Herbal.* Rochester N.Y.: Healing Arts Press, 1994.

Harper-Shore, Lt. Col. F. *Medicinal Herbs.* Essex, England: Daniel Compa, 1952.

Hobbs, Christopher. *Women's Herbs, Women's Health.* Loveland, CO: Interweave Press,1998.

Hoffman, David.*The Herb User's Guide. The basic skills of medicinal herbalism.* Northhampshire, England: Thorson's Publishing Group, 1987

_____.*The New Holistic Herbal.* Rockport, MA: Element Publishing, 1993

Bibliography

Hopman, Ellen Evert. *A Druid's Herbal*. Rochester, VT: Desti Books, 1995

Hurley, Judith. *The Good Herb*. New York, NY: William Morrow, 1995.

Kamen, Betty. *Hormone Replacement Therapy, Yes or No*. Novato, CA: Nutrition Encounter, 1996.

Kamm, Minnie Watson. *Old Time Herbs for Northern Gardens*. New York, NY: Dover Publications, 1938.

Kenner, Dan, and Yves Requena. *Botanical Medicine*. Brookline, MA: Paradigm Publishing, 1996.

Kloss, Jethro. *Back to Eden*. Santa Barbara, CA: Woodbridge Press, 1975.

Lark, Susan. *Anemia and Heavy Menstrual Flow*. Los Altos, CA: Westchester Publishing Co., 1993.

_____. *Menstrual Cramps*. Los Altos, CA: Westchester Publishing Co., 1993.

Levy, Juliette de Bairacli. *Nature's Children*. New York, NY: Warner Publications, 1972.

Lonsdorf, Nancy. *A Women's Best Medicine*. Los Angeles, CA: Jeremy Tarcher, Inc., 1993.

Lu, Henry C. *Chinese Herbal Cures*. New York, NY: Sterling Publishing Co., 1994.

Lust, John. *The Herb Book*. New York: Bantum Books, 1980.

Marion, Joseph. *The AntiAging Manual*. South Woodstock, CT: Information Pioneers, 1996.

McGuffin, Michael, et al. *Botanical Safety Handbook*. Boca Raton, FL: CRC Press, 1997.

Miles, Karen. *Herb and Spice Handbook*. Norway, Iowa: Frontier Cooperative Herbs, 1989.

Mowry, Daniel. *The Scientific Validation of Herbal Remedies*. New Cannan, CT: Keats Publishing, 1992.

Murray, Michael. *The Healing Power of Herbs: The Enlightened Person's Guide to the Wonders of Medicinal Plants*. Rockland, CA: Prima Publishing, 1992.

Ody, Penelope. *The Complete Medicinal Herbal*. New York, NY: Dorling Kindersley Publishing, 1993.

Onstad, Dianne. *Whole Foods Companion*. White River Junction, VT: Chelsea Green Publishing, 1996.

PDR for Herbal Medicines. Montvale, NJ: Medical Economics Company, 1999.

Peterson, Lee Allan. *A Field Guide to Edible Wild Plants.* Boston, MA: Houghton-Mifflin, 1977.

Robertson, Diane. *Jamaican Herbs. Nutritional & Medicinal Values.* Kingston, Jamaica: Jamaican Herbs Limited, 1990.

Royal, Pen C. *Herbally Yours.* Provo, Utah: BiWorld Publications, 1978.

Scalzo, Richard. *Naturopathic Handbook of Herbal Formulas.* Durango, CO: Kivaki Press, 1993.

Shannon, Marilyn. *Fertility, Cycles and Nutrition.* Cincinnati, OH: Couple to Couple League, International, 1996.

Schar, Douglas. *The Backyard Medicine Chest.* Washington, D.C.: Elliot & Clark Publishing, 1995.

Semler, Tracy. *All About Eve.* New York: NY, Harper Collins Books, 1995.

Stansbury, Jill. *Botanical Medicines Acting on the Female Reproductive System.* American Herbalists Guild, 8th Annual Symposium Proceedings, 166-92.

Stone, Gaynell. *Languages & Lore of the Long Island Indians.* Suffolk Co., NY: Suffolk County Archeology Society, 1980.

Swerdlow, Joel. *Nature's Medicine.* Washington, DC: National Geographic, 2000.

Tantaquidgeon, Gladys. *Folk Medicine of the Delaware and Related Algonkian Indians.* Harrisburg, PA: The Pennsylvania Historical and Museum Commission, 1995

Tenney, Louise. *Today's Herbal Health.* Provo, Utah: Woodland Books, 1982.

Tierra, Michael. *Planetary Herbology.* Santa Fe, N.M.: Lotus Press, 1988.

Twitchell, Paul. *Herbs, The Magic Healers.* Menlo Park, CA:IWP Publications, 1971.

Weed, Susan. *Healing Wise.* Woodstock, NY: Ash Tree Publications, 1989.

——————. *Breast Cancer, Breast Health!* Woodstock, NY: Ashtree Publishing, 1996.

Werbach, Melvyn and Michael Murray. *Botanical Influences on Illness.* Tarzana, CA: Third Line Press, 2000.

Zampieron, E. and Kamhi, E. *The Natural Medicine Chest.* New York, NY, M. Evans, 1999.

About the Author
and Contributors

Ellen Kamhi, Ph.D., R.N., *The Natural Nurse* (www.naturalnurse.com), is the coauthor of *The Natural Medicine Chest* (M. Evans) and *Arthritis, The Alternative Medicine Definitive Guide* (alternativemedicine.com). She is a professional member of the American Herbalists Guild (AHG), is nationally board certified as a holistic nurse (HNC), and is on the advisory board of the *International Journal of Integrative Medicine*. Dr. Kamhi has been involved in the field of Natural Medicine for over thirty years. She attended Rutgers and Cornell Universities, and sat on the panel of traditional medicine at Columbia Presbyterian Medical School and holds appointments as Clinical Instructor at the Department of Family Medicine, SUNY at Stony Brook Medical School. She is on TV and radio nationally, and along with media partner, Eugene Zampieron, N.D., leads ecotours for cures to indiginous areas worldwide. Ellen Kamhi practices holistic medicine, with Serafina Corsello, M.D. She is a consultant to the herb industry and a frequent speaker at conventions nationally.

Steven Angel

Steven Angel, B.A., D.C., has been actively involved in researching the healing power of sound and music for over twenty-five years. Dr. Angel has presented his research to the First International Conference on Holistic Health and Medicine in Bangalore, India in 1989. Dr. Angel is the founder and director of the Angel Holistic Healing Center located in Long Beach, New York, where he teaches about vibrational medicine in the form of sound and music therapy, light/color therapy, homeopathy, nutritional counseling, non-force chiropractic, cranial-sacral therapy, massage therapy, and reflexology. Dr. Angel is completing the book, *Man, Music, and Infinity*. He can be reached at Angel Holistic Healing Center, 2-12 West Park Ave., Suite 201, Long Beach, NY, 11561; 516-889-6462, www.chirosonics.org.

Serafina Corsello

Serafina Corsello, M.D., F.A.C.A.M., is the founder and executive director of the Corsello Centers for Integrative Medicine in Manhattan, New York. She is an internationally respected clinician, lecturer, and the initiator and cofounder of the Foundation for the Advancement of Innovative Medicine (FAIM). Dr. Corsello was one of the twenty-five physicians who in 1992 participated in the formation of the Office of Alternative Medicine within the National Institutes of Health. She is the author of *The Ageless Women*. She can be reached at the Corsello Center for Complementary Medicine, 212-399-0222, www.corsello.com

Kristina Louise DeMarco

Kristina Louise DeMarco, R.N., M.S., is a certified adult health nurse practitioner; She joined the Corsello Centers for Nutritional and Complementary medicine in 1995 and worked with Dr. Serafina Corsello as her mentor with expertise in female hormonal balancing and general integrative medicine. She coauthored with Ellen Kamhi "Infertility; an Integrative Approach," which was published in the *International Journal of Integrative Medicine*, July 2000.

Shauyon Liu

Sharon Liu, O.M.D., offers a traditional Chinese medicine formula based on the herbs mentioned in this book designed specifically for women going through menopause. She has also designed several other Chinese herbal formulas. She is a licensed acupuncturist trained as an M.D. in China. Her offices are located at 1331 Stony Brook Road, Stony Brook, NY, and at 1 West 34th Street in New York City. Call for more information on Chinese herbal formulas: (631) 689-6221; in New York City call (212) 868-0145.

Glen Rein

After receiving a Ph.D. in biochemistry from the University of London, Dr. Rein pursued an orthodox biomedical research career for twenty-five years at a variety of prestigious academic institutions. In 1988, he left academia to pursue his interest in energy medicine and founded the Quantum Biology Research with a research grant from the Fetzer Institute. Since then he has been characterizing new forms of energy which are involved with the natural healing process. Dr. Rein is the author of the book *Quantum Biology: Healing with Subtle Energy* and has published over thirty articles in top biomedical journals and books. He has lectured internationally and has made numerous media appearances on radio and TV. He can be contacted at quantumbio@att.net.

Eugene R. Zampieron

Eugene R. Zampieron, N.D., A.H.G., is a licensed naturopathic physician, professional herbalist, and medical botanist specializing in the non-toxic treatment of autoimmune and rheumatological disorders, especially arthritis and fibromyalgia. He received his Bachelors degree in biological and marine sciences from S.U.N.Y. at Stony Brook, and his doctoral degree in naturopathic medicine from Bastyr University of Natural Health Sciences in Seattle, Washington. He is a professional member of the American Herbalist Guild.

Dr. Zampieron also acts as a botanical formulations inventor and natural products consultant. He is a syndicated radio and multimedia host, magazine columnist, and co-executive of Natural Alternatives Health, Educational, and Multimedia Services, Inc. He is a professional speaker who lectures audiences internationally. Along with business partner Ellen Kamhi, Dr. Zampieron has written *The Natural Medicine Chest* (M. Evans) and Arthritis, *The Alternative Medicine Definitive Guide* (Alternativemedicine.com). He has also been quoted in Rodale Books, as well as hundreds of articles. The duo also produce several syndicated radio programs and appear on TV often to discuss aspects of natural medicine.

Dr. Zampieron has spent much time over the last twenty years apprenticing, researching, and documenting the ethnobotany and spirituality of the Maroon and Rastafarian people of Jamaica. He cohosts one of the longest running Reggae music shows in America, *Rockin' Irations*, and is coexecutive with Dr. Kamhi of EcoTours for Cures, which leads educational vacations and botanical eco-exursions into the rainforests around the globe.

Dr. Zampieron was involved with the founding advisory board of the first naturopathic medical college on the east coast in over 100 years—the University of Bridgeport College of Naturopathic Medicine. Here he serves as an adjunct assistant professor of clinical medicine currently teaching the doctoral students botanical medicine, pharmacognosy, and ethnobotany. He practices and resides in Connecticut and lives on a ten-acre woodland preserve with his wife Kathleen and children Caitlin and Kevin. He hikes, wildcrafts herbs, and gardens organically. Contact him at 800-829-0918, ezkpz@juno.com.

Index

Index

garlic, 19, 24
gastrodia elata. *See* tain ma
gemstones, 176
gentian, 173
ginger, 183
  and breast compress, 51, 54, 115
  and digestive problems, 13
  and love potion, 61
  and pregnancy, 46
  and Zingiber Zing, 115
Ginger Tea, 46,115
Ginkgo biloba, xvi
glandular functions, 118
glucose, 2
glycosides, 91, 105, 139, 154
Glycyrrhiza glabra. *See* licorice root
goat milk, powdered, 55
gobo. see burdock
goldenseal, 24, 46, 82
gorse, 173
gotu kola, 184
Grandpa's Pine Tar Soap, 12
green beans, 6, 182
green cardamom, 115
green foods, 10, 181, 182, 183, 184
  leafy vegetables, 29
  and libido, 59
  and mini-fasting, 20
  and nursing, 53
  and pregnancy, 49
  and raisiHg progesterone, 33
  tea, 45, 83
  and xenoestrogens, 31
gymnena sylvestre, 26

hair growth, 72, 181
hands-on healing, xvii
hawthorne berries, 26
he huan pi, 72
headaches, 106, 182
  and castor oil packs, 100
  and dandelion, 107
  and dong quai, 109
  and motherwort, 132
  and nettle, 134
  and premenstrual syndrome, 25
  and rose buds, 142
  and Saint John's wort, 146
  and tain ma, 72
  and yeast infections, 22

healing skin salve, 81
Healthy and Natural Journal, 187
Healthy Green Beans, 117
heart, 182
  and ginger, 114
  and motherwort, 70, 132
  and stress, 30
  and yuan zhi, 72
helonis dioica. see false unicorn root
hemorrhoids, 52, 121
hemp, 12
hepatitis, 128, 130
Herbal Gram Magazine, 187
herbal
  knowledge, xvi
  medicine, xv
  oil, 85
  teas, 77
  therapies, xx
herbicides, 2, 9, 28, 29
herbs, xix
  and fertility, 41
  and menstruation, 16
  purity of, 87
  quality of, 87
  and stocking compress, 83
Heritage Products, 64
herpes, 128
high blood pressure. see blood pressure
hijiki. see sea vegetables
Hildebrandt, Gunther, 166
HIV, 128
ho shu wu, 181, 182, 183, 184
  and fertility, 41
  and liver, 20
holistic medicine, 67
Holt, Stephen, 196
holy signatures, xvi
hops, 6, 31, 51, 53
Horizon Herbs, 188
hormone replacement therapy (HRT), 67
hormones, xix, 5, 38, 68, 186
horse chestnut, 47, 184
hot flashes, 182
  and black cohosh, 69
  and burdock, 96
  and chaste tree berry, 70
  and menopause, 66

Index

Index

and nursing, 53
and premenstrual syndrome, 26
mimulus, 173
minerals, 107, 136
mini-trampoline, 32
Miso Soup, 149, 153
Mitchella repens. see partridge berries
monk's pepper. see chaste tree berry
monoamine oxidase (MAO), 147
moods, 3, 72. *See also* irritability
and menopause, 66
and premenstrual syndrome, 25
and Siberian ginseng, 155
morning sickness, 114, 140, 158, 183.
See also nausea
mother's cordial, 94
motherwort, 181, 182, 183, 184
and hot flashes, 70
and pregnancy, 50
mouth ulcers, 141
Muria Puama, 62
muscle
aches, 91
mass, 2, 72
relaxation, 5, 84, 126
music, 169, 171
musk, 64

National Formulary, 106
Natural Alternatives, 9
Natural Medicine Chest, 85
natural therapies, xvii, 25, 27, 41
Nature Conservancy, 9
Nature's Answer, 24, 47, 188
nausea, 114, 183. *See also* morning
sickness
nerve pain, 146
nervousness, 105, 106, 132
nettle, 70, 181, 182, 183, 184
and breast compress, 54
and lymph system, 21
and nursing, 53
and nutritional support, 10
and pregnancy, 45, 50
New Living Magazine, 70, 188
niacin, 140
night sweats, 67
nipples, sore/cracked, 54
nori. see sea vegetables
North American Menopause Society, 65

nursing, 5, 183
nutritional support, xvii, 10, 38, 53, 59

oak, 173
oatmeal, 47, 52, 83, 96
Oatmeal Smoothy Facial, 137
oats, 181, 182, 183, 184
and libido, 59
and love potion, 61
and nursing, 53
oatstraw, 4849
okra, 19, 52
olive oil, 81, 122
omega-3 oils, 12, 32, 45, 69
onion, 19, 153
oregano, 24
oregon graperoot, 82, 93
organic foods, 19, 29, 31
orgasm, 58
Original Swiss Aromatics, 188
osteoporosis, 67, 72, 183
ovarian cysts, 99, 100, 158, 183
ovaries, 2, 4, 5, 136
ovulation, 3, 4, 5, 40
oxytocic, 49

pain, 181
and ginger, 114
and Jamaican dogwood, 124
and kava kava, 126
and nettle, 134
and yan hou su, 159
palm of Christ. see castor bean plant
Panax ginseng, 62
parasites, 76
parsley, 19
partridge berries, 94
patchouli, 64
Pausinystalia yohimbe, 63
Peony, 110
peppermint, 13, 46, 83
peptic ulcers, 128
perimenopause, 66
perineal compress, 50
peristalsis, 98
Pert, Candace, 172
Peruvian ginseng, 62
pessary, 82
pesticides, 2, 9, 28, 29

Index